THE COMPLETE GUIDE TO
INDOOR ROWING

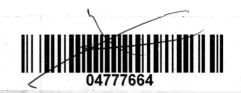

THE COMPLETE GUIDE TO

INDOOR ROWING

Jim Flood and Charles Simpson

BLOOMSBURY

LONDON · BERLIN · NEW YORK · SYDNEY

Note
While every effort has been made to ensure that the content of this book is as technically accurate and as sound as possible, neither the author nor the publishers can accept responsibility for any injury or loss sustained as a result of the use of this material.

Published by Bloomsbury Publishing Plc
50 Bedford Square
London WC1B 3DP
www.bloomsbury.com

First edition 2012

ISBN 978 1 4081 3332 3

Acknowledgements
Cover photograph © Getty Images
Inside photographs © Grant Pritchard unless otherwise specified and excluding the following: pp. 146, 147, 157 courtesy of Concept2, chapter 10 photographs provided by case subjects.
Illustrations by David Gardner
Designed by James Watson
Commissioned by Charlotte Croft

This book is produced using paper that is made from wood grown in managed, sustainable forests. It is natural, renewable and recyclable. The logging and manufacturing processes conform to the environmental regulations of the country of origin.

Typeset in 10.75pt on 14pt Adobe Caslon by Saxon Graphics Ltd, Derby

Printed and bound in China by C&C Offset Printing.

CONTENTS

INTRODUCTION

Rowing machines have been used in gymnasia for over 100 years but the last 10 years have seen a huge growth in the number of people using them. This phenomenon is associated with the growth of fitness centres and the modern desire for an athletic body shape, a combination that rowing machines in particular have benefited from.

So why is the rowing machine proving to be so popular? The answer is probably a result of the smooth 'feel' of the rowing action, the low impact on the limbs and the large range of muscles that are exercised. For the many people who suffer from knee problems that limit their ability to run or to exercise, it is an ideal solution.

There is increasing evidence that exercise can help in the treatment of depression. Exercise helps people to improve their confidence and self-image, gives them positive goals and releases endorphins, the hormones that induce feelings of well being. It can also improve sleep and reduce stress. Rowing machines are easy to use and provide an ideal introduction to an exercise programme for beginners.

Relieving stress though exercise is also a useful process for men and women in the armed services. In many of the fortified camps used by the coalition forces in Iraq and Afghanistan, rowing machines are used to provide intensive exercise in places where space is at a premium. Another place where space is at a premium and it is necessary to exercise is on the International Space Station, where a rowing machine is used by astronauts to maintain fitness and bone density.

Rowers have been using rowing machines since the late 70s both for fitness training and to develop good technique. When rowers had to train on rowing machines because of dangerous conditions on the water, this inevitably led to competitions over set distances – much like regattas only using rowing machines instead of boats. This soon developed into a separate sport based on competitions using rowing machines.

Indoor rowing competitions began in the United States and quickly spread. The British Indoor Rowing Championships is now the largest participatory indoor sporting event in the UK. In 2010, throughout the world:

- 40,000 athletes competed in indoor regattas;
- 400 indoor rowing events were staged in 40 countries; and
- 1900 athletes competed in the World Indoor Rowing Championships.

There are many more smaller competitions organised by fitness centres and schools. For example, in 2010, over 7000 students in 20 schools in County Durham (UK) took part in a Get Going, Get Rowing competition. In London in 2011, over 2500 students between the ages of 14 to 18 took part in an indoor rowing event organised by London Youth Rowing. In both of these examples, the vast majority of the participants were from state schools – a point worth emphasising because in the UK, junior rowing on water is still dominated by private schools.

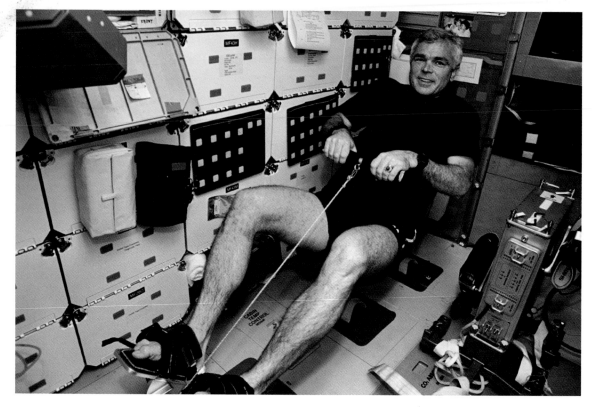

Fig 0.1 Astronaut Michael R. (Rich) Clifford, mission specialist, uses the rowing machine temporarily deployed on the Space Shuttle Endeavour's mid-deck. Many of the crew members put in time on the device during the week and a half mission (courtesy of NASA with permission)

For competitions it is necessary to have a standard machine which is the Concept2 rower. The key factor is a display unit that can be programmed to ensure that competition between participants is absolutely fair. For example, if rowers set the drag lever at different settings, the microprocessor in the display unit will still calculate how far they travel with each stroke.

New technologies have opened up the possibility of virtual competitions. You can now hook up your Concept2 machine to a computer and compete against other rowers thousands of miles away. You can also check your fitness levels against tables of results and obtain advice on training and technique.

WHAT THIS BOOK AIMS TO ACHIEVE

This book has been written as a resource for individual rowers, coaches and trainee coaches. Because it is in the format of a resource, it is not necessary to read the chapters in sequence. Find the sections that interest you and make this a

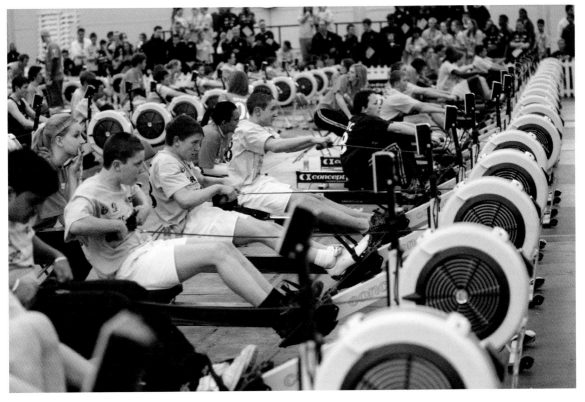

Fig 0.2 Competitors in the 2010 British National Junior Indoor Rowing Championship (courtesy of London Youth Rowing with permission)

starting point to explore further. We have aimed to provide basic information that can be used as a resource for beginners, as well as detailed advice and analysis on technique and training.

We believe that skilled coaching is vital so chapter 4, which covers coaching styles and techniques, is important to us. You might not be a coach but this section should enable you to have informed discussions with your coach about the style of coaching that suits you best.

Sport now draws on the sciences of physiology, biomechanics, nutrition and psychology, and our work draws on the latest research in these fields.

We have aimed to provide a basic grounding in these areas so that you will have a basis for more advanced study.

We have included case studies on individual rowers. We hope that you will be able to identify with, and learn from, some of their thoughts and experiences. They are of different ages and backgrounds – a reflection of the broad base of society from which indoor rowers are drawn. Several of them are senior citizens, proving that age is no barrier to this sport. In fact the benefits of exercise for those over 50 are now well recognised, and indoor rowing provides a low impact form of exercise, making it an ideal system for this purpose.

Indoor rowing has also been quicker than most sports to provide opportunities for the participation of people with disabilities. Adaptive rowing events have been included in competitions since 2004, another aspect of the inclusive nature of this sport.

If you are using a rowing machine to train for rowing, then you will find much useful information that will help with your technique and training. Using a rowing machine is not just about getting the highest score possible – you can use it to improve your speed on the water through better technique.

Therefore, whatever level of experience you have with indoor rowing, and whatever it is you hope to achieve, we hope that this book will help to support and promote your development in this sport.

THE DEVELOPMENT OF INDOOR ROWING

Rowing machines have been in use for about 140 years. The first patent was filed in the United States in June 1871 by WB Curtis. Between 1871 and 1952 there were more than 40 patents filed for rowing machines. One of the best known was the Narragansett hydraulic rowing machine designed in 1900 and manufactured until the late 50s. They were installed in the gymnasium of the Titanic, the ship that hit an iceberg and sank on its maiden voyage in April 1912, and there is a short sequence in the 1997 film which shows Narragansett rowing machines in use.

Rowing machines were also used in hospitals for rehabilitating the injured. A 1938 news film documenting a rehabilitation centre at the Albert Dock Hospital in London shows seamen who are recovering from injuries using rowing machines that move across the floor.

It is likely that the development of rowing machines was influenced by rowing races that attracted large numbers of spectators in both London and New York. By 1715 there was an established annual race between the Thames Watermen who operated the ferry services around the rivers of London. The winner was awarded a coat and badge, and this event is still held today, making it the longest continuously recorded

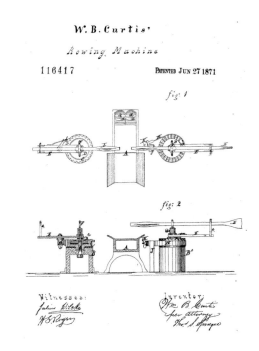

Fig 1.1 WB Curtis' rowing machine, the first patent for such a machine, in 1871 (courtesy of US Patent Office)

sporting event in the world. By 1756 there were rowing races in New York that created a great deal of public interest. All of these races were for prize money so this form of the sport could not be considered a 'gentlemanly' activity. However,

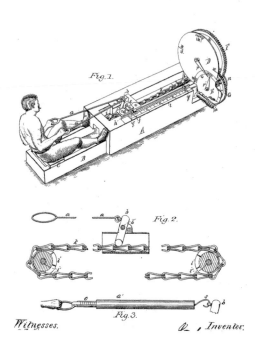

J. H. TROWBRIDGE.
MACHINE FOR EXERCISING AND DEVELOPING THE MUSCLES OF MANKIND.

No. 282,589.   Patented Aug. 7, 1883.

Fig. 1.

Fig. 2.

Fig. 3.

Witnesses.   *Inventor.*

Fig 1.2 Another rowing machine patent, from 1883: 'A machine for exercising the muscles of mankind' (courtesy of US Patent Office)

rowing for pleasure was a 'gentlemanly' activity, and one which is described in Jerome K Jerome's novel *Three Men in a Boat*, published in 1889.

Another influence on the development of the rowing machine is likely to have been the cult of physical fitness amongst 'gentlemen', which began in the mid 1800s. Newspapers of the day carried adverts for a range of patent devices for exercising muscles.

The early rowing machines were designed to simulate the rowing action and to provide an opportunity to maintain fitness indoors. In this sense, they are the forerunners of the huge range of fitness machines that are now available. These early rowing machines had fixed seats, much like the boats they were modelled on. A much later development was the sliding seat that enabled rowers to take a longer stroke. This is thought to have originated when Thames Watermen greased their seats so that they could slide up and down on them.

From the 1960s the coaching of rowing became based less on intuition and more on evidence from accurate testing, therefore, there was a need for a machine that could accurately measure the force that rowers could exert, and also the level of fitness they had achieved. This is now known as evidence-based coaching. A more detailed description of the methods of testing can be found in chapter 8.

This need for testing stimulated the development of a new breed of rowing machines that could provide accurate data and would be a useful training aid. One of the first of these was developed in Australia in the early 40s and, using the Greek words for work (ergon) and measure (metron), it was given the name 'ergometer'. The three people involved in this development were Frank Cotton, Professor of Physiology at Sydney University, John Harrison, an engineer, and Ted Curtain, a welder and boilermaker. Frank Cotton believed that in rowing (and in other sports) there was too much emphasis on style. He wanted a machine that would prove that fitness and power were much more important factors. John Harrison, a successful surf rower, was tested on an early version of the ergometer which indicated that he had huge potential as a flat water rower. This proved to be the case when he rowed for Australia in a coxless four at the 1956 Olympics. Both John Harrison and Ted

Curtain made significant contributions to Frank Cotton's first machine to provide the basis of the modern ergometer – and a system for objective research into fitness and power. John Harrison was offered a lectureship in mechanical engineering at the University of New South Wales where he completed a PhD in 1966 on the design of a universal ergometer. Rowers will be interested to know that he is also credited with the development of the big blade and the use of computer-aided design to develop modern racing boats. He also predicted that an ergometer would not be able to accurately represent the action of rowing in water until it had a fixed seat with a moving footrest. Several of the machines developed by Cotton, Harrison and Curtain were built in and used in rowing clubs in Australia. One of these machines has survived and is in the collection of exhibits at the River and Rowing Museum at Henley on Thames in the UK.

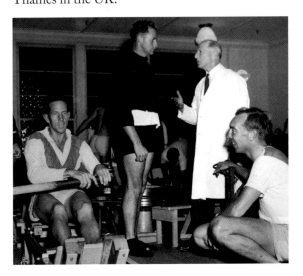

Fig 1.3 The first ergometer. Professor Frank Cotton is in the white coat (courtesy of Leichhartd Rowing Club, Sydney, Australia)

A version of this Australian machine was exported to the United States and used in the selection process for the 1968 Olympic rowing team. This machine was developed further by the Gamut Engineering Company of California and used extensively in rowing training in the United States throughout the 70s.

However, what enabled the sport of indoor rowing to develop was the adoption of the

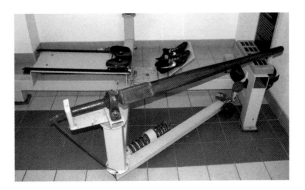

Fig 1.4 A Gamut ergometer on display at Florida Institute of Technology (courtesy of Florida Tech Athletics)

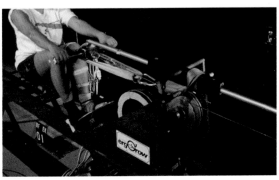

Fig 1.5 Another machine that provided valuable research data in the 70s was the Gjessing ErgoRow (courtesy of Professor Gordon E. Robertson of the School of Human Kinetics, University of Ottowa)

Concept2 as a standard machine that enabled comparisons to be made across all rowers. The range of Concept machines was developed by Peter and Dick Dreissigacker, two brothers who were both very successful rowers. Dick Dreissigacker rowed for the USA in the 1972 Olympics. In 1980, after establishing a successful company for the design and development of oars, they decided to diversify into other products. After considering such items as masts for windsurfers and ski poles, they eventually decided to develop a training machine for rowers that would be cheaper than the Gamut or the Gjessing models that cost around $3000 at that time. Their first prototype was made from bicycle parts. This quickly developed into the first production model, costing $600. The market need was quickly established with an order for 20 of the Model A machines for Columbia University, which were fitted with a bicycle computer to provide a measure of speed and distance. A significant breakthrough was made with the Model B, which was fitted with a display unit that gave much of the information that is now seen on the latest PM4 display units, such as split times and set workouts.

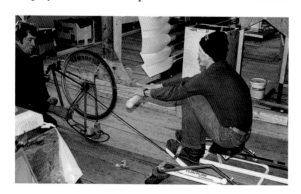

Fig 1.6 The first prototype Concept rowing machine (courtesy of Concept2)

This turned it into a much more sophisticated training machine that could be used to monitor individual progress, as well as a means of fair testing athletes for their potential as competitive rowers. Concept2 machines are now the accepted standard for competitions – and for use in rowing clubs throughout the world.

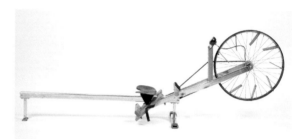

Fig 1.7 The first production Model A Concept rowing machine (courtesy of Concept2)

THE DEVELOPMENT OF NATIONAL AND INTERNATIONAL COMPETITIONS

By 1982 a group of ex international and Olympic rowers known as the Charles River All Star Has-Beens (C.R.A.S.H.-B.) was organising competitions using rowing machines provided by the Dreissigacker brothers. This grew into the World Indoor Rowing Championship, although it is still affectionately known as the CRASH-B. There are now national and local competitions held in most countries that participate in international rowing events.

In 2010, at the 20th British Indoor Rowing Championship (BIRC) there were over 2200 competitors. The oldest (who set a world record) was 100 years of age.

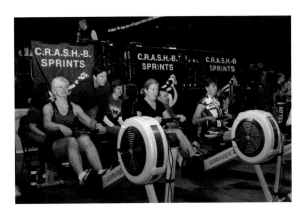

Fig 1.8 The C.R.A.S.H.–B. sprints (courtesy of C.R.A.SH.–B)

Today, there are also many indoor rowing sports events that are not based on racing over a set distance. Many clubs and organisations now use rowing machines for fund-raising events and challenges. They also offer fitness classes in which activities take the form of non-competitive games.

COMPETING OVER THE INTERNET

It is now possible to compete against another person on your rowing machine without ever leaving your home. Using a combination of a computer, a connection to the Internet, software such as Skype and a webcam, you can link up with others to organise your own race.

ADAPTIVE INDOOR ROWING

This is a sport that developed from the wider movement to provide access to indoor rowing for people with different forms of disabilities.

The first adaptive sports competition for those with disabilities was in 1924 in Paris. The Silent Games was a version of the Olympic Games for deaf people. After the Second World War there were rehabilitation programmes for injured soldiers

and civilians involving games that were adapted from various sports. In 1948 the Olympic Games was held in London, during which a wheelchair Olympics was held at Stoke Mandeville hospital. This movement gradually resulted in the modern Paralympic Games that now runs in parallel with the Olympic Games. There are also adaptive competitions in several other World Championship events. It is possible that, in the future, indoor rowing might become an Olympic event.

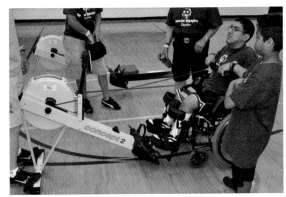

Fig 1.9 Adaptive events organised by UcanRow2 in the United States (courtesy of UcanRow2)

There are now adaptive categories in some indoor rowing events. One such category is for wheelchair users. This requires a wheelchair to be in a fixed position in front of an adapted Concept2. The use is limited to arms only or arms and body.

One very interesting development is that the sport of indoor rowing is opening up to people with spinal cord injuries (SCIs), which cause paralysis of the lower part of the body. Using a system called Functional Electrical Stimulation (FES), muscles can be stimulated through electrodes on the surface of the skin which then cause paralysed limbs to move in a set sequence –

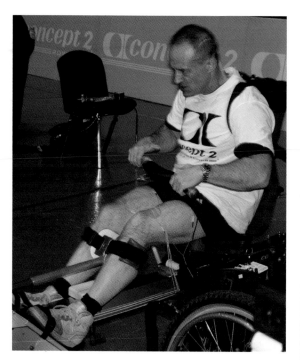

Fig 1.10 Robin Gibbons, a champion FES rower (courtesy of Robin Gibbons)

such as that of the leg action needed to operate a rowing machine. Since 2004 there has been an FES section in the British Indoor Rowing Championship (see Robin Gibbon's case study, p. 153).

Rowing machine systems that supply exercise for paralysed limbs can provide enormous benefits such as improved fitness and blood circulation, which can help to avoid diabetes and respiratory disease.

Although indoor rowing is a sport that began with rowers using rowing machines as part of their training programmes, the rate of growth has been such that there are now more non-rowers than rowers taking part – and certainly more people using rowing machines than rowing on water.

Summary

- Indoor rowing, as a competitive sport, is growing rapidly
- Rowing machines have been used for over one hundred years but it is only in the last 30 years that a standard machine has been developed that is suitable for competitions
- Internet technology means that individuals and groups can compete against each other in any part of the world where Internet access is available
- Rowing machines can be modified easily for use by adaptive athletes.

HOW ROWING MACHINES WORK

2

This chapter explains some of the basic mechanisms and technology used in rowing machines. The main purpose of a rowing machine is to simulate the action of rowing with an oar in the water. For example, when the oar is placed in the water at the beginning of the stroke, the boat is driven forward through the water by pushing with the legs and pulling on the handle. At the end of the stroke the oar is extracted from the water and moved forward for the next stroke. Good rowing machines simulate the 'feel' of this action. Even the best machines provide only a limited simulation and the search continues for a machine that will give exactly the same feel of an oar in the water. For the sport of indoor rowing this is not essential, but as a tool for training rowers, it is much more important.

CREATING RESISTANCE

There are five basic methods for creating resistance (i.e. imitating water resistance) on the handle of a

> ### Keypoint
> A rowing machine aims to simulate the action of an oar in the water.

rowing machine when an athlete gets into position and begins to row.

1. A MECHANICAL BRAKE

The simplest method, found on low cost rowing machines, uses a wheel with a form of brake which slows the wheel down, and which can be adjusted to change the force required to spin the wheel. This is similar to the system used on many static cycling machines. It was also used on the original Gjessing machine mentioned in chapter 1.

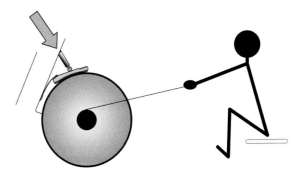

Fig 2.1 Brake mechanism

The cord is wound around a pulley which has a free wheel recoil mechanism similar to that of a starting cord for an outboard motor or petrol powered lawnmower. This provides a very poor 'feel' for the rowing action because the wheel slows down quickly between strokes causing a heavy load at the beginning of the stroke.

2. HYDRAULIC RESISTANCE

This was popular in some of the early designs such as the Gamut machine mentioned in chapter 1. The system is still used on compact designs for home use.

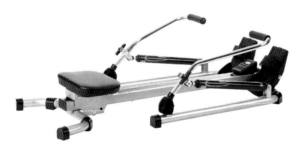

Fig 2.2 The Beny improver dual hydraulic rower (courtesy of Beny Fitness Equipment)

The resistance is provided by hydraulic cylinders that have the appearance of bicycle inflaters. These 'inflaters' are filled with oil which provides a steady resistance as the piston moves through it. The piston is fitted with a one-way valve that provides resistance in the drive phase but hardly any resistance in the recovery phase.

3. THE AIR IMPELLER

This is in fact an air pump that is in wide use both in the home and in industry. The most obvious examples that can be found are the hairdryer and vacuum cleaner. Both are devices for blowing air, which is what happens in the Concept2 machines and others that use the same system.

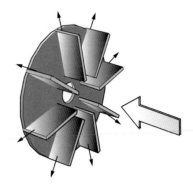

Fig 2.3 The impeller

As the impeller spins, the air is moved away from the centre by centrifugal force. As the air moves away from the centre, more air is drawn in to replace it. This effect can be felt by holding a book or magazine at the bottom edge and flicking it around like a fan.

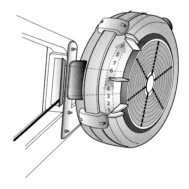

Fig 2.4 The damper lever that changes the effort required to row on the machine

In the case of a hairdryer, the air being forced to the periphery of the impeller is captured by a casing and is directed out through a nozzle. With rowing machines that use this system the air is allowed to escape through small holes around the perimeter of the impeller casing. By restricting the amount of air that can enter at the centre of the impeller, less air is pumped and less effort is required to spin the impeller – which is what happens when you move the 'damper' lever to a lower number. When the damper lever is set to a higher number the size of the air intake increases, more air is pumped and consequently the work load increases.

> When you watch an action movie in which someone falls from the roof of a tall building, the stunt person is actually attached to a rope which is wound around a pulley that drives an impeller used in some rowing machines. By adjusting the damper, the speed of descent is controlled. The film of the event then needs to be speeded up to show a realistic rate of fall.

This system does give a reasonable 'feel' of an oar in the water. However, there are differences; the loading on the feet and the back is greater than it would be in a boat. There is a deeper analysis of this in chapter 8.

4. THE WATER ROWER SYSTEM

This system is used on some of the most stylish looking machines with the frame being made of polished wood. The resistance to the handle is provided by a cord and pulley, similar to the recoil system used in the mechanical brake wheel system. The pulley drives a rotating paddle inside a small water tank. The paddle churns the water around in a similar manner to a washing machine. The resistance can be altered by increasing or decreasing the amount of water in the drum – not a quick or easy method compared to other systems.

There are strong claims that the water rower system gives a more realistic feel of an oar in the water but there is an absence of quantitative results to confirm this.

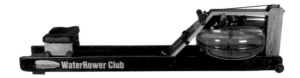

Fig 2.5 The Water Rower (courtesy of WaterRower)

5. THE MAGNET SYSTEM

This is based on the principle of magnetic braking. A recoil system spins a flat segmented disc made from copper or a copper/aluminium alloy. As the

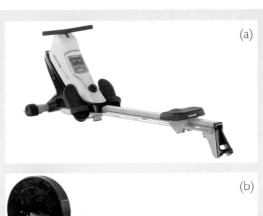

Fig 2.6 (a) Kettler CoachE; (b) There are now many budget rowing machines on the market of which the Artemis II Air rower is one example. (courtesy of Fitness-Superstore/Kettler and Beny Sports UK)

fins of the disc pass between magnets, eddy currents are generated that slow the fins down. As the fins pass the magnets at greater speed, the braking effect increases. These machines tend to be compact, quiet and very low cost compared to other systems. They are useful for general fitness training but are rarely used by serious athletes.

THE FLOATING HEAD ROWING MACHINE

Rowing in a boat has a different feel from that of a standard rowing machine. This is partly because the boat is moving at the same time as the rower – and in particular the foot stretcher is moving relative to the rower.

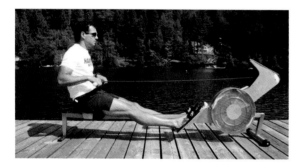

Fig 2.7 The Rowperfect rowing machine (courtesy of Ursula Grobler/Carlos Dinares, www.rowperfect3.com)

The floating head rowing machine is an attempt to recreate a more realistic 'feel' of the oar in the water. The foot stretcher is fixed to the impeller unit and slides with it. As the rower begins the drive phase both the seat and the impeller unit slide apart. This can be quite disconcerting after using a conventional rowing machine, however, there is some evidence that scullers in particular can benefit from using the floating head system.

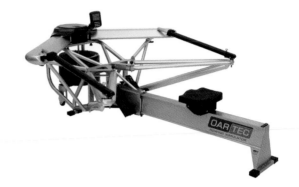

Fig 2.8 The Oartec Rowing Simulator, one of the latest machines, which aims to provide a realistic feel for both sculling and sweep oar rowing (courtesy of Oartec)

COMPUTERISED TECHNOLOGY

'How well am I doing?' is a question that any user of a rowing machine will want to ask at some point. Most good systems now have a digital display that will provide a wealth of information. Within a given time, you will want to know the 'distance' you have travelled. You might want to be able to 'count down' to a specific distance or time – that is you can pre-set the display to show the remaining distance or time in which you have to complete the session. Also you might want to know the rate you are rowing at – that is the number of strokes per minute. The feedback provided by a digital display is a vital tool for monitoring your training.

Keypoint

For many indoor rowers, one of the key elements of the display is the split time for 500m.

RATE (STROKES PER MINUTE)

The rate meter works by a magnet on the seat passing over a fixed sensor, which is a coil of wire. As the magnet passes close to the coil it induces a current to flow – and it is this small pulse of electricity which is counted in terms of strokes per minute.

DISTANCE

The distance is measured in terms of the number of turns of the flywheel – also by a magnet passing a coil. A bicycle computer uses the same system.

DRAG

As the damper setting is changed to make it easier or harder to row, the 'drag factor' can be displayed on the screen. This is important in competitions or tests in which the drag factor needs to be the same for all competitors. The most accurate measurement of the drag factor is found in the impeller system in which a pressure sensor inside the impeller casing is related to the speed of rotation. Simply setting the damper to the same settings on different machines is not accurate enough for fair testing.

The Concept2 PM 4 display has a wide range of display options including the ability to connect machines together for a competition that shows the progress of several 'boats'. It can also be connected via a computer to the Internet to race against competitors on the other side of the world.

Summary

- Rowing machines are designed to simulate the action of rowing on water
- Even the best machines are unable to replicate the exact 'feel' of rowing on water – but they are constantly improving
- The display unit is a key component that shows the speed and distance rowed, and, therefore, how hard the rower has been exercising. Currently display units on different machines are not compatible in terms of results – but this might become possible in the future to compare performances on different machines.
- The cheaper range of rowing machines are useful as basic home exercise machines.

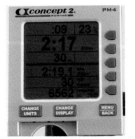
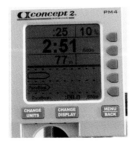
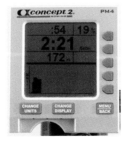
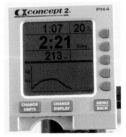

Fig 2.9 The Concept2 PM4 display

EFFECTIVE TECHNIQUE

3

This chapter outlines the importance of good technique and posture at different points in the stroke cycle. Good technique not only improves your performance, it helps to avoid undue strain and injury.

Your aim might be to use the rowing machine to improve your general health and fitness, you might wish to enter indoor rowing competitions or you might be using the rowing machine as part of your training for rowing. Whatever your aims, it is important to understand the importance of making effective use of the large muscle groups. Chapter 5 will explain physiology in greater detail, but the first point to be clear about is that rowing on a rowing machine is mainly a matter of pushing with the legs rather than pulling with the arms. You will still hear people talking about a 'strong pull', when in fact they should be saying 'a strong push'! So, when using a rowing machine, think 'push', not 'pull'.

> **Keypoint**
> Indoor rowing is a pushing sport, not a pulling sport.

THE CORRECT KINETIC CHAIN

It is obvious that the muscle groups in your legs are much larger and more powerful than those in your arms, so it is sensible to make effective use of them. Think about the position you adopt if your are asked to do a standing jump: without really thinking about it, you crouch down then drive your body upwards using the power of your legs (you might also swing your arms to help with the balance). From the crouching position to the point where your feet leave the ground, your muscular skeletal system has moved through a series of positions called a kinetic chain. As very young children we learn to use a series of kinetic chains to be able to walk, run and jump.

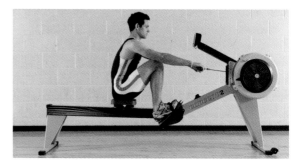

Fig 3.1 The beginning of the drive phase

Unlike running or jumping, using a rowing machine is not a natural action so it is necessary to learn the correct kinetic chain, that is the sequence of movements, that will maximise your effort.

THE DRIVE PHASE

We'll begin at the point where you start to push with the legs. This is known as 'the catch' – the point at which you would catch hold of the water if you were rowing in a boat. It is also the beginning of the drive phase of the stroke cycle. At this point in the kinetic chain, the shins are vertical, the back is straight and leaning forward, the head is upright and the arms are long and loose. It is helpful to check your position using a large mirror, or if you don't have one to hand, ask a friend to stand to the side of you.

back straighter if you set the heel position to the lowest point. Also only move forward to the point where your back is reasonably straight, even if your shins are not vertical.

If you are using a rowing machine for the first time, we suggest that you try slow short pushes with the legs so that you feel the pushing action. Stay in a forward-leaning position and resist the temptation to pull with the arms. Think of your arms as chains and your fingers as hooks.

Important
Avoid strain and injury by developing good posture and by maintaining the damper lever on a low setting.

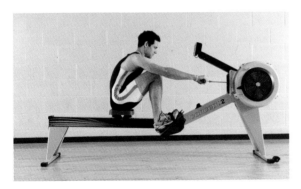

Fig 3.2 An example of a weak kinetic chain

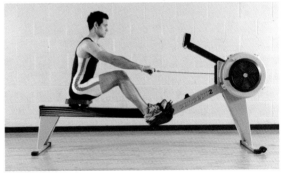

Fig 3.3 Good posture in the drive phase

Now it might be the case that, even trying as hard as you can, your kinetic chain at this point looks more like the picture above. This could be because of a lack of flexibility or a habitual tendency to sit in a slumped posture – so try a bit harder as this particular kinetic chain position can lead to back strain! You will be able to get your

Gradually push further back so that you are moving backwards and forwards in a comfortable forward-leaning position. When you can move backwards to the point where your legs are straight, you are ready for the next part of the kinetic chain.

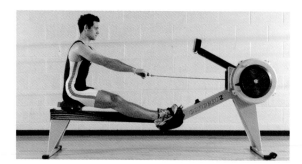

Fig 3.4 Spine in line with the pelvis

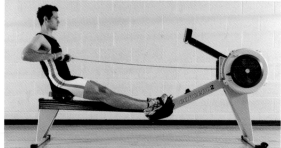

Fig 3.6 The end of the drive phase

It is important to maintain the forward-leaning position until your legs are straight. Resist the temptation to heave the shoulders back in an attempt to pull harder – this will break the effective kinetic chain.

And finally the arms come into use to draw the handle close to the chest. This is the completion of the drive phase of the rowing stroke.

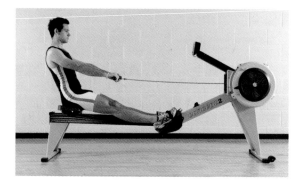

Fig 3.5 Swing back from the hips

In the drive phase think about pushing with the legs, 'hanging' off the handle with straight arms and keeping the back straight (not curved). Swing the shoulders backwards only after the hands have passed over your knees.

THE RECOVERY PHASE

The next stage is the recovery phase, well named because it is a chance to recover from the effort that has been put into the drive phase.

The back swings from the forward-leaning to the backward-leaning position using the lower part of the pelvis as the pivot point.

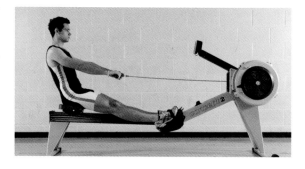

Fig 3.7 The beginning of the recovery phase

Stage 1 of the recovery phase is simply to move the hands smoothly away from the finish position close the to chest until they are fully extended.

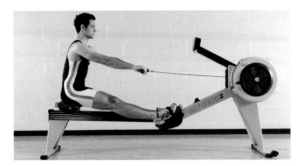

Fig 3.8 Swing forward from the hips

Think of the recovery phase as the preparation for the drive phase.

Next the body swings or rocks over into the position for the catch. The knees should not lift until the hands have passed over the top of them. Unless you are remarkably flexible, you will feel considerable tension in the back of your legs at this point. Remember that this is the recovery phase so it is important to be relaxed but with sufficient tension in the lower back to maintain good posture.

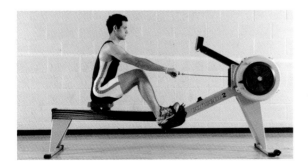

Fig 3.9 The trunk is already in the catch position

When your hands have passed over your knees, your knees lift up – but not before! A good check is to ensure that you feel your hamstrings stretching before you allow the knees to lift.

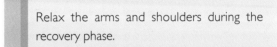

Relax the arms and shoulders during the recovery phase.

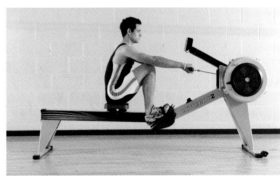

Fig 3.10 Squeeze forward until the shins are vertical

As you reach the point of the catch, slow down and compress your chest up to your thighs in a controlled way. If you reach the catch still travelling at speed, the effect will be to bounce back, placing considerable strain on your joints and muscles.

Our friend with the poor posture has to curl his back over to reach forward for a long stroke, and also the point of pivot at the end of the stroke is likely to be above his pelvis rather than below it. The aim is to have a 'neutral spine' throughout the stroke; that is a straight spine in line with the pelvis.

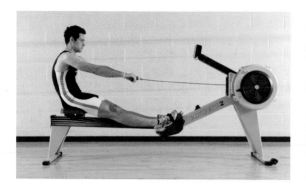

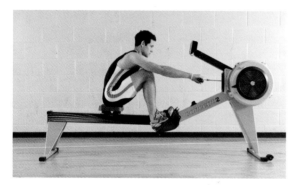

Fig 3.11 Examples of poor posture

RATIO AND RHYTHM

The ratio is the difference in the time spent during the drive phase and the time spent during the recovery phase. If you watch inexperienced rowers, they will move up and down the slide at the same speed. To work effectively over long periods you need to spend at least double the amount of time over the recovery phase (and to practise relaxing) so that you limit the build up of lactic acid in the muscles. One way of achieving this is to count to a steady beat of one, two, three. One beat is for the drive phase, and two beats for the recovery phase. Practise also using a four and five beat count in which the drive phase is completed to one beat. The rhythm is the measure of your ability to maintain a consistent

number of strokes per minute. Rowing in a rhythmic manner will help you to get into the 'zone' – a feeling that you can row for long periods without exhausting yourself.

Establishing a good rhythm is the basis of a good performance.

COMMON FAULTS TO IDENTIFY IN YOUR OWN POSTURE AND TECHNIQUE

OVERREACHING

Watch for the shins going forward beyond the vertical position which reduces the power of the first part of the drive phase. This is known as 'overreaching', and is common in people with a lot of flexibility. Raising the height of the heel cups can help to correct this problem.

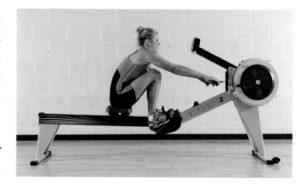

Fig 3.12 Overreaching

LOSS OF POWER IN THE LEGS

Being in an upright (vertical) position at the catch with the back vertical causes a loss of power in the legs due to an inefficient kinetic chain. Watch also for people who begin the stroke leaning forward but then swing into the vertical position too early – which results in the same problem.

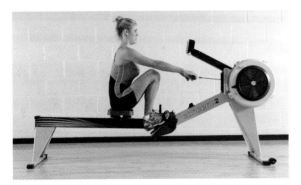

Fig 3.13 Too upright

BACKWARDS-LEANING POSTURE

This is a more extreme version with a backwards-leaning posture. It is very common to notice this in fitness centres where people using the ergo have received no training.

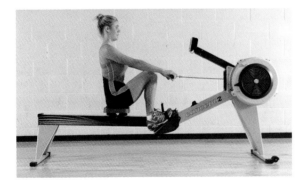

Fig 3.14 Shoulders swing back too early

BENT ARMS

This looks like a good position until you notice the bent arms. If the arms are bent when they take

the load, it causes considerable tension around the neck and shoulders, again causing a loss of power because of a poor kinetic chain.

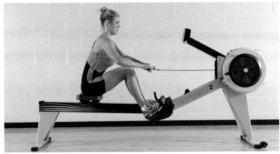

Fig 3.15 Rowing with bent arms

'BUM SHOVING'

This form of kinetic chain is known very unkindly as 'bum shoving'. It happens at the catch when the hips accelerate backwards faster than the shoulders.

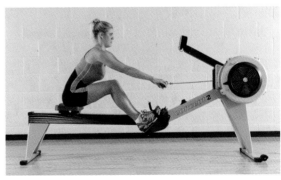

Fig 3.16 Pushing the hips back before the body moves

Your aims are to:

- row with a smooth flowing movement with the correct kinetic chain at each point in drive phase;

- feel that you are pushing back through the hips, not the shoulders;
- relax during the recovery phase and move at least half the speed of the drive phase;
- slow as you compress the chest up to the thighs as you approach the catch and
- be aware of the importance of good technique in order to avoid strain or injury.

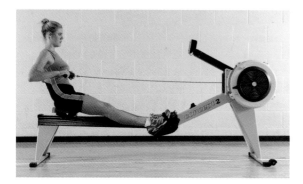

Fig 3.17 Linking all the parts together in a smooth action

Fitness is about being able to maintain good posture for longer.

REFINING YOUR TECHNIQUE FURTHER

Establishing a basic technique is the first step; the next step is to be fit enough to be able to maintain it for longer periods. You will have heard a commentator on sports events talk about competitors 'losing their shape' as they get tired. Typically, the head drops and the body loses stability and control as the muscles tire or begin to seize up. To develop your own technique it is important that you are able to maintain your 'shape' (that is the correct kinetic chain) so, initially, it is important that you do not exercise beyond the point where this deteriorates as a result of tiredness. Initially, aim for longer slower sessions rather than short fast ones. Check your posture in a mirror and/or work with a partner so that you can check each other.

You should also aim to have the support of an experienced coach who will help you to refine your technique by designing a fitness programme for you, improve your posture through stretching exercises and monitor your progress. Everyone is slightly different and a good coach will help to adapt the basic technique to the physiology of the individual.

USING THE ROWING MACHINE FOR COACHING ROWING SKILLS

This section is aimed mainly at coaches and athletes who use rowing machines to develop skills for rowing on water. However, the exercises will also be of benefit to indoor rowers.

There are several challenges that interact when coaching athletes on the water to improve their rowing skills. These include the following:

- Environmental conditions such as wind and disturbed water can place constraints on the athlete's ability to respond to instructions.
- Less experienced athletes find it difficult to maintain perfect balance – which makes it difficult to maintain a constant stroke pattern.
- In a crew boat, slight differences in technique can be a cause of instability.

- It is not always easy for the coach to be close enough to the athletes to communicate well.

> The rowing machine provides a stable platform for the coach and athletes to analyse and improve posture, and to practise skills.

Many rowing coaches include coaching sessions on the rowing machine as an essential process in the development of skilled rowers. Up close and personal to a rower, a coach can provide better feedback on some of the subtle skills of rowing.

In the drive phase this includes:

- good drive off the balls of the feet and suspension off the handle;
- the seat moving in synchronicity with the hands and shoulders;
- good acceleration of the handle right through to the finish;
- arms long and loose; hands holding the handle very lightly and using the fingers as hooks – with the wrists and top part of the hands kept in line with the arms; and
- elbows 'zipped' back and shoulder blades squeezed together for a strong finish.

In the recovery phase this includes:

- good sequencing of the hands, body and slide at the beginning of the recovery;
- good posture, keeping the trunk and head still moving towards the catch;
- relaxed arms and shoulders right up to the point of the catch;
- deceleration as the catch is approached;
- squeezing up to the catch so that the impression is that the knees are meeting the chest – rather than the chest dropping on the the knees; and
- head kept still and vertical throughout the stroke.

Many rowing clubs have mirrors in training room so that athletes can observe themselves and work at correcting weaknesses in technique.

One of the roles of a coach is to set up experiences so that the athlete feels the desired effect. Learning a correct action by feeling it is much more powerful than simply being told. This is known as a kinaesthetic learning experience.

> Being able to feel when an action is correct is a sign of good progress.

What follows is a series of exercises that coaches commonly use to provide kinaesthetic learning experiences for their athletes.

TRAJECTORIES

The trajectory of different points of the body is one of the keys to achieving good rowing technique on the water. For example, the trajectory of the shoulders is horizontal throughout the stroke, apart from a slight arc as the body swings over at the end of the drive phase and then when the shoulders follow the hands at the beginning of the recovery phase.

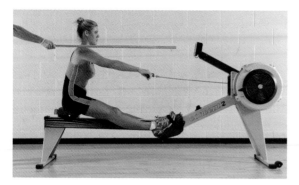

Fig 3.18 Following a guide for the correct shoulder trajectory

Any tendency to overreach at the catch, or rotating the shoulders back too early in the drive phase will result in a change of trajectory. If the athlete practises following a stick held horizontally at shoulder height by the coach or partner, this can help to improve their posture.

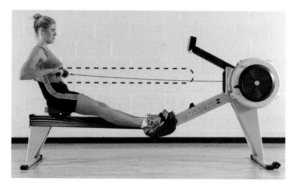

Fig 3.19 Trajectory of the hands when rowing in a boat

The trajectory of the hands is also important to place the blade (oar) in the water at the catch, and to extract it at the finish. The hands lift up at the catch and tap down at the finish. Between these points it is essential for good balance that the hands move horizontal to the water. Athletes are often told by coaches to imagine that they are drawing their hands over the surface of a table in the drive phase and returning the hands under the table in the recovery phase. This action is not easy to achieve on a rowing machine because the chain emerges from a fixed point. Following this trajectory is something to try in practice and not when trying to achieve a good score.

When analysing the trajectories of the shoulders and hands, it can be appreciated that the arms have to rotate at the shoulder joint to avoid lifting when the shoulders begin to swing back. When rowing in a boat it's important to keep the neck girdle (shoulder area) relaxed so that the arms can rotate slightly to compensate for the trunk rocking over. A lack of rotation causes the hands to lift and consequently the blade to go too deep. A similar problem can occur if the trunk swings back too early in the drive phase.

ROWING ON A SLOPE

Rowing on a slope can provide two important kinaesthetic learning experiences. One is that athletes can feel more easily the effect of pushing with the legs and hanging (suspending) off the blade handle at the catch.

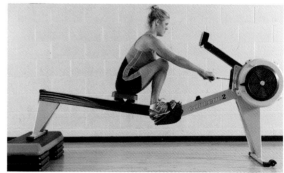

Fig 3.20 Ensure that this is set up in a safe and stable manner

The other key point relates to approaching the catch, which needs to be done in a controlled manner. Coaches can often be heard to call 'Stop rushing into the catch'. Rushing into the catch causes a loss of control and precision in placing the blade in the water. It also saps energy as the legs have to act as brakes to slow the body down, and then suddenly change direction. Rowing on a slope exaggerates the feeling of rushing into the catch and enables the athletes to learn to control it.

FIXING THE HANDLE IN POSITION

The handle is fixed in position with a strong strap attached to the handle and a fixed part of the rowing machine. Because the athlete has to drive against this until they lift off the seat, it is vital to protect against the possibility of injury caused by

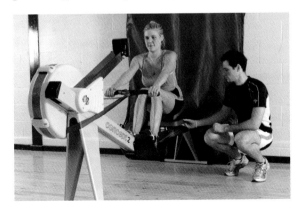

Fig 3.21 The handle is fixed in position with a strong strap

the strap slipping or breaking. One way of doing this is to back the rowing machine against a wall with a crash mat in place to absorb the potential impact.

As the athlete lifts up, the seat will slide forward, so it also useful to have another person to hold the seat in place during the suspension.

The exercise of the athlete driving with the legs until they lift off the seat to a height of around 10cm can provide two different kinaesthetic learning experiences:

1 The feeling of hanging off the blade handle at the catch.
2 The feeling of the effect of squeezing the glutes (the gluteus maximus muscles).

Recent research has shown that significant improvements in performance can be achieved if athletes learn to use their glutes in conjunction with the leg drive. The exercise is to hold the position for 30 seconds at a time, concentrating on using the glutes rather than the legs to achieve the lift – and at the same time keeping the shoulders relaxed. The exercise can be repeated at later stages in the drive phase by lengthening the retaining strap that holds the handle in a fixed position.

A further use of the fixed handle is to provide a feel for the difference in the drive force that occurs if the angle of the back changes. What is needed is an industrial type of spring balance, to weigh up to 200kg, that can be attached in place of the retaining strap. The effect of having the back upright or collapsed over will show a dramatic reduction in the force that can be applied. This also provides a demonstration of the importance of a good kinetic chain.

PUSHING BACKWARDS THROUGH THE HIPS

There is a common tendency for athletes to drive backwards through the shoulders rather than the hips – a tendency that causes the shoulders to move backwards ahead of the hips. The 'feel' for driving through the hips can be provided by the athlete sitting on the rowing machine without holding the handle, and by providing some pressure against the lower back to push against. The easiest way to provide this is to work in pairs with one athlete providing the resistance with hand pressure on the lower back. It is good practice to hold a folded towel or cushion against the lower back to avoid the potential discomfort of athletes feeling that they are being touched in an intimate manner.

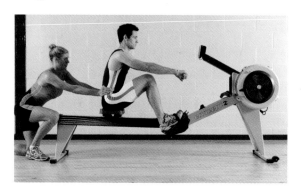

Fig 3.22 Rowing without holding the handle

The person applying the pressure to the lower back should be able to feel a difference when the rower concentrates on using his or her glutes.

MAINTAINING CONTACT WITH THE FOOTSTRETCHER

This exercise is about maintaining some downwards pressure through the feet at the end of the drive phase when the body swings back and

the feet tend to lift. Watch a person rowing strongly on a rowing machine and the chances are that you will notice the feet lifting against the straps towards the end of the drive phase and the beginning of the recovery phase. This is not critical in the case of indoor rowing, indeed, it is necessary for the athlete to pull themselves forward against the foot straps. The problem is that in a boat, a similar action can cause problems with the balance as it is more difficult to keep the body stable when there is no downwards pressure on the footstretcher. In fact, with the main body weight hanging from the shoes (boats have fitted shoes rather than straps) the body can act as a pendulum. There needs to be good control at the three points of contact with the boat: the blade handle, the seat and the footstretcher. If contact with the footstretcher is lost, the other two points of contact also tend to suffer from instability – which is then transmitted to the boat.

> **Tip**
> Wearing thin-soled shoes when using a rowing machine (instead of thick-soled trainers) can improve the feel of pushing off the ball of the foot.

One exercise is to use the rowing machine without strapping the feet in. This can be scary at first as athletes can topple over backwards – so initially one person standing behind to prevent this is a sensible safety measure. However, what this exercise does promote is the use of the head to maintain balance. Inclining the head slightly forward at the end of the stroke prevents the toppling back effect and maintains contact with the footstretcher.

Rather more fun can be provided by setting a challenge. The challenge is to hold two pieces of folded paper under the ball of the foot – and to row with increasing pressure. The folded pieces need to be set at about 45 degrees from the vertical so that if released by lack of foot pressure, they fall sideways. It helps if the athletes are told to point their toes at the finish of the drive phase.

MAINTAINING THE TRIANGLE

When rowing in a boat, the triangle formed by the hands, shoulders and seat should stay constant between these two points in both the drive and recovery phases. There will be a slight change in the shape of the triangle as the hands lift at the catch and tap down at the finish. In effect this is difficult to achieve on a rowing machine because the hands tend to follow the downward line of the chain. However, it is an important coaching point that can be demonstrated.

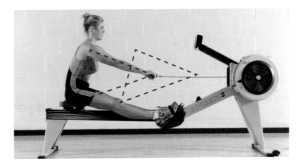

Fig 3.23 Maintaining the triangle between these two positions

Summary

The rowing machine is an excellent tool for reinforcing skills taught on the water, especially as it provides a stable platform for analysing and correcting problems with technique. It also provides the coach with close analysis of the subtle changes that can be made to suit the style and physiology of different athletes.

COACHING STYLES AND TECHNIQUES

4

Most of us have been fortunate to have experienced a good coach or a good teacher. The particular qualities are difficult to define – but we know when we experience it! A good coach gives you the confidence to believe that you can succeed, explains things in a way that makes sense, yet also challenges and motivates you to do better. So how do you, as a coach, create those feelings in your athletes?

One way of considering this question is to identify the qualities of a poor coach. Rowing, along with many other sports, has a tradition of coaches behaving like dictators, often referred to as the 'command model' of coaching. Coaches who follow this model expect to be obeyed without question, are motivated through fear and criticism and tend to appear bullying and abusive in the way they communicate. However, some of these coaches have been spectacularly successful, so it is not a quality that can be completely ignored. It is in fact a method that has tended to work well with elite athletes who have become inured to the method and who are able to resist the negative effects.

> Coaching is about telling, selling and succeeding.

Most coaches of indoor rowing will be working with beginners and improvers with a wide range of athletic abilities. In this case, the role of the coach is to provide an introduction to the activity that is enjoyable, gives participants the feeling that they are making progress and which will make them want to come back for more. The role of the coach is to build confidence through a progression of activities in which a level of success can be achieved by each participant. Coaching is not simply providing instruction; it is about planning, analysing, providing feedback, ensuring safe practice and facilitating progress. It is about enabling individuals to achieve much more than they could on their own. With this in mind, it is useful to think about the stages of learning a skill and of the techniques that can be used to facilitate the learning process.

THE THREE STAGES OF LEARNING A SKILL: PREPARATION, PRACTICE, AUTOMATIC

PREPARATION

The preparation phase is one in which participants are taking on board a lot of information and a new set of skills that they are trying to fit together. An effective strategy for this stage is to separate out the parts of the strokes into actions that are easily carried out, easily remembered and then gradually linked together to form the whole stroke.

If you are coaching a first session then you might begin with a brief demonstration of the whole stroke, by someone with good technique, to show participants the ultimate goal. Then begin by teaching small sub-sections of the stroke that can be gradually linked together.

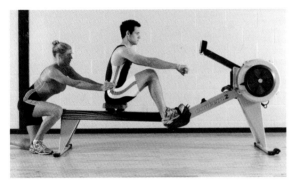

Fig 4.1 Feeling the effect of pushing back with the legs without using the handle

For example, a good starting point is to introduce the idea of rowing being a 'pushing' rather than a 'pulling' sport. This is helpful to the participant because it reduces the number of things to think about and feel. Think about not using the handle but replacing it with a piece of wood of similar size and shape, then the participant only has to feel how to push back with the legs.

It's useful to have participants working in pairs with one on the rowing machine and one observing

and assisting. In this case the observer can, with permission, provide some resistance to the push back at the point shown. The observer can also help the participant to maintain the correct posture (straight arms, back inclined forwards) during the push back. When this is being achieved reasonably well, the use of the handle can be included. The next step could be to work on the end of the drive phase in isolation.

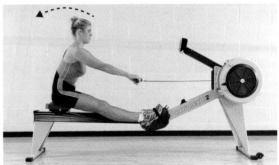

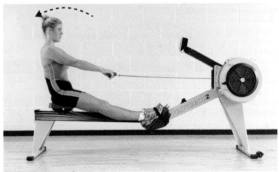

Fig 4.2 Swinging the body back at the finish

The next sub section or part of the stroke to isolate could be the first part of the recovery phase.

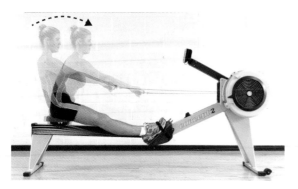

Fig 4.3 Swinging the body forward at the recovery

It can be useful to reinforce a sequence like this by giving the actions numbers, for example: 1 hands away, 2 body over, 3 legs released and the seat moves forward. You can often hear this sequence being called by coaches who are working with highly experienced rowers – it is a point that needs constant reinforcement.

> Instructions and explanations should be short – and followed quickly by activity.

During this preparation stage it is important to give the participants experience of linking the sub-sequences together – but also to go back to practise these in isolation until the whole sequence can be performed smoothly and confidently. When this is achieved, the participants are moving on to the 'practice stage'.

PRACTICE

The practice stage (sometimes referred to as 'the grooving stage') is where the participants understand the skill and can perform the sequence. What they need is lots of repetition and feedback

to fix the sequence in place. Coaching during this stage is a process of gradual improvement through feedback.

It is important during the preparation and practice stages that participants experience success by having targets that are realistic and achievable for them as individuals. Playing games can relieve the boredom factor at these stages and provide for a degree of fun. Most of the display units will have a games section in the menu.

AUTOMATIC

The automatic stage is one where the participants have learned the subroutines and can put them together in a smooth flowing movement, almost without having to think about it. At this point it is possible to concentrate on improving levels of performance through training programmes that you discuss and agree with individuals.

COMMUNICATION: THE FOUR Ps (POSITION, PROJECTION, PACE AND PITCH)

Good communication with groups is a key skill in coaching. The four Ps provide some basic guidelines for good practice – and for projecting your personality and enthusiasm.

POSITION

Always position yourself so that the whole group can see you and any equipment that you are using. For example, if you are demonstrating an aspect of technique, it is essential that everyone has a good view – so you might have to arrange the seating (or standing!) with this in mind. Face to face contact with all the group is vital for good communication.

Also it enables you to monitor their reaction and watch for signs that they might not have fully understood what you are explaining. You can then check with questions and, if necessary, offer an alternative explanation.

Many coaches use overhead projectors or PowerPoint slides to demonstrate their coaching points. Here are a few golden rules on how to present information in this way:

- The overhead projector, and the video projectors that have largely replaced them, which are used to show PowerPoint slides, were designed so that the presenter can maintain face to face contact with the audience. Avoid the practice of turning your back on your audience and reading from the screen (a very common mistake).
- Reading directly from the slides is also poor practice because most people can read seven times faster than you can speak – so give comments that amplify the key points.
- Follow the rule of no more than three points per slide.
- Use a minimum 18 point font size so it is legible from the back of the room.
- Use as few words as possible – keep your points succinct and to the point.

PROJECTION

Some of your good teaching will be lost if there are members of the group who are unable to hear you, so **project** your voice and check that everyone can hear easily. If not, you might have to bring the group closer to you.

PACE

Think about the **pace** at which you are unloading information. Too much information too fast and you might 'lose' your audience. Too little too slow and they might become bored. Plan with the composition of your group in mind, and be prepared to change in response to their reaction. Breaking up an idea into parts (for example, the parts of a stroke) and gradually linking them together, can enable a group to cope with a faster pace. Regular summaries of key points will also help your group to stay with you. Remember also the importance of scheduled breaks – and to finish on time.

PITCH

There is nothing worse to listen to than a boring monotone voice, so ensure that you use your voice in an expressive manner. One of the ways to achieve this is by changing the **pitch** of your voice. Other ways include changes in modulation, slight pauses and the speed of your delivery. Watch and listen to how news reporters make use of their voices and body language to emphasise key points.

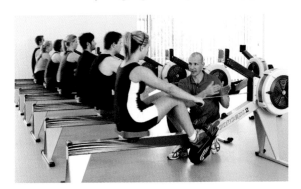

Fig 4.4 Coaching a technical point (courtesy of Concept2)

Be confident in expressing your own personality when coaching.

FEEDBACK – CLOSING THE LEARNING LOOP

As a coach, you have a very clear idea in your mind of what you want the participants to know and do. You can ensure that you have transmitted the information to the participants but how do you check that what is in their minds bears any similarity to what is in your mind? What methods can you use to improve this communication, and what methods can you use to check that their understanding is similar to yours? This process is known as 'closing the learning loop'.

> As a coach you need to know what your aims are and how you will close the learning loop.

Let's begin with the first part of the process. People learn in different ways so, in explaining what you want participants to do, aim to use a range of different verbal and visual means of communicating. Aim to provide kinaesthetic experiences, for example, ask participants to feel their legs doing the pushing. Make use of analogies and visualisations. For example:

- Think push not pull.
- Float forward in the recovery phase.
- Listen for the wheels on your seat slowing down as you approach the catch.
- Feel the handle accelerating towards you in the drive phase.
- The rowing action is like weight lifting turned through 90 degrees.

Clearly one way of checking that your explanation has been understood is to see the results, so be quick with praise and encouragement when your input produces the desired output. Be prepared to use different modes and methods of explanation when the desired output is not achieved. Aim to think of the failure to achieve the desired output as a failure of your explanation, rather than a failure of the learner to understand.

As well as explaining 'what' and 'how', explain 'why'. If learners understand the reason for doing something, they are more likely to achieve it. For example, 'Lean forward more at the catch – because this will provide a good kinetic chain enabling you to produce a more powerful leg drive.' The 'because' part of the explanation provides a good reason to do it – and is also a memory hook to aid retention. Better still, give a demonstration of this effect.

> Learning is a collaborative process between the coach and participants.

One obvious way of closing the learning loop is to summarise key points at the end of the session and to ask questions. Avoid asking questions of the whole group; ask questions of individuals by name. Better still, ask them to group into pairs and compare their thoughts about what they have learned during the session, then feedback the points to you as the coach. This is a very good check on how effective your teaching has been – and it gives you a further chance to correct any misunderstandings.

> Participants in coaching sessions are nearly always trying hard to achieve what the coach wants. If this is not being achieved, a good coach will assume that it is her or his fault.

Video is a very effective way of providing feedback. Often athletes do not really understand that their posture is poor until they see themselves on video. Elite rowers often have training sessions on rowing machines, wearing goggles with mini screens inside so that they see a side view of themselves in real time.

BE RESPONSIBLE FOR YOUR OWN PROFESSIONAL DEVELOPMENT

As a coach you need to be both a life-long learner and a thief. Completing a coaching qualification is only the beginning. You need to think regularly about how you can improve your own performance. Analyse the reasons for why a particular method or technique worked well or did not work at all. What can you learn that will influence how you plan future sessions?

Watch other coaches in action and steal their ideas – but develop them further so that they become your own. Share your ideas with other coaches; there is nothing like talking about an idea to get a better understanding of it.

PARTICIPANT-FOCUSSED COACHING

The training of coaches in most sports in the UK is now based on the concept of 'participant-focussed coaching'. This is a concept that is part of the policy of the of the United Kingdom Coaching Certificate (UKCC) framework for coaching qualifications. All coaching qualifications, including the Level 1 and Level 2 Indoor Rowing Coaching Certificate, are based on this methodology. This is part of a much wider trend. For example, doctors are now encouraged to view their patients as clients, and as active participants in decisions to be made about the treatment that might be required. So what does this mean for you as a coach? Here are some guidelines to think about:

- Be friendly and welcoming at the initial meeting. The individuals you are about to introduce to indoor rowing are likely to be quite nervous and anxious about what is required of them. Aim to put them at their ease with an 'icebreaker' activity (see p. 30).
- Establish how they wish to be referred to, individually and collectively. Referring to a group of women as 'guys' as in 'Okay, guys, let's make a start', can create barriers to communication unless it has been agreed first.
- Briefly outline the programme for the session (plus mandatory safety points about emergency exits, etc.) and make it clear that if there is anything that they do not understand, it is likely to be your fault for not explaining it clearly enough, so they should not hesitate to ask for clarification. Remember that there is a strong tendency for people to nod their heads in answer to questions like 'Is that clear then?' They prefer to answer in the affirmative rather than to appear to be stupid. Use the 'lollipop stick' method of asking questions to ensure an inclusive approach (see p. 31).

- Think about how to make best use of 'open questions' and 'closed questions' (see p. 31).
- Begin with small easy steps. At subsequent sessions, always begin with a review and practise what took place last time. Think of better ways to check that the participants are feeling comfortable other than by asking 'Are you all okay doing this then?' For example, try asking individuals, 'Tell me what you are finding easy, and what you are finding a bit more difficult.'
- Plan to break the session up into a series of 'chunks'. Explain the purpose of each chunk and give a brief review at the end of each one.
- Be responsive to the different progress of individuals – and aim to be fair in your distribution of individual tuition.
- Be generous in your praise and encouragement – and always find something positive to say before being constructively critical. There is very clear evidence that participants are much more willing to listen to constructive criticism if they hear something positive first. Even experienced learners who know what to expect still want to hear the positive points first.
- Cabin staff in aircraft are trained to say 'Would you put you seat upright for me?' That last bit of the request 'for me' has proven to be much more effective in producing a positive response. Try it!
- Think about asking participants to work in pairs and to help each other to achieve the objectives you have set. Asking participants to try explaining an action to someone else is an effective way to improve their own understanding.
- If it is absolutely necessary to touch someone in order to explain a point (and this should be a last resort), you must ask their permission in private first.

ICEBREAKER ACTIVITIES

These activities are designed to get people talking so that they participate in discussions and answer questions more readily. A very simple one is to ask people to pair up with someone they do not know (or do not know well). Set them 5 minutes to find out about their interest or motivation for attending the course. After 5 minutes, link the pairs into fours and, in turn, get them to introduce their first partner to the other two – and outline their interest or motivation for attending the course.

This form of pairing up is useful when posing questions. For example, if you ask, 'Why do we say that rowing is a pushing sport, not a pulling sport?', you will generate much better answers by asking pairs to discuss the answer rather than by posing the question to the whole group.

EXAGGERATION

When asked to achieve a strong position with the arms or body an athlete does not always get it right first time. Sometimes exaggerating the advice can result in the desired position being achieved. For example, if you want an athlete to incline their body forward at an angle of about 10 degrees, and this proves difficult to achieve, ask for an angle of 30 degrees – and he or she might just get it right.

KINAESTHETIC LEARNING

This is learning by feeling. Feeling when an action is correct is so important when learning a new sport. As a coach, aim to get your athletes feeling what is happening. For example, feeling the pressure through the ball of the foot as the legs begin the drive phase, or feeling the arms long and loose in the recovery phase.

THE 'LOLLIPOP STICK' METHOD OF QUESTIONING

The name comes from the technique of asking everyone to write their name on a lollipop stick. The sticks are then placed in a jar. Each time a question is asked, the teacher draws a lollipop stick out of the jar and that is the name of the person who is asked the question. When the jar is empty the sticks are replaced for the next round of questions. Cards work just as well as lollipop sticks.

This method avoids a few people becoming dominant in the questioning process, and ensures that everyone has the opportunity to answer questions, even though some might wish to avoid them. This method also tends to make individuals think about the answers because their name might be on the card.

OPEN AND CLOSED QUESTIONS

Closed questions require a simple one word or very short specific answer. An example would be, 'Chris, can you tell me what the maximum setting is on the damper lever?' An open question requires an explanation, for example, 'Sam, how do we set the drag factor on the display unit?'

Answering closed questions first, is a way of checking that basic facts are understood. It is also a way of establishing confidence within the group that their answers will not be ridiculed – which is always a fear of a group of learners with a new coach. Open questions are much better at checking the understanding of processes and concepts and of providing feedback on the need for further teaching inputs.

GAMES AND CHALLENGES
On the rowing machine

Games and challenges can add variety and interest to both leaning technique and training on the ergometer. There are several games on the PM4 Display Monitor that are worth exploring as a means of adding variety.

Naming the parts

The objective is to name the main parts of the rowing machine correctly. Provide each small group with a set of name cards for the main components. The task is to match each card to the correct component by placing it on top or close to it.

Ergo golf – for four to six participants

A target distance is set, say 500m. In turn each member of the team takes one stroke only. The winner is the team to finish closest to the target distance.

First to the split

The coach calls out a split time for 500m (usually a slow time for the group). The first person to hold the split time for five strokes is the winner. This needs an independent observer for each machine.

Rowing to music

The music needs to have a rhythm that is easy to follow on the rowing machine. Also, placing the machines in a circle facing inwards can help the 'aerobic class' effect. Ask each person in turn to take the lead as the music tracks change.

WHAT DO PARTICIPANTS FEEL LIKE IN A PARTICIPANT-FOCUSSED COACHING ENVIRONMENT?

Often 'not very comfortable' is the answer! Beginners often come to indoor rowing with experience of other learning environments in which the teacher or trainer takes complete control. The only responsibility that the learner has is to listen to an explanation and repeat the desired action. It can come as a shock to the system when learners are expected to participate in their own learning and the coach is behaving more like an 'adviser on the side, rather than a sage on the stage'. Pause for a moment and think about your own experience of this kind of learning.

'What do you feel about what you have learned this session?' is the kind of question that can produce a stunned silence unless the participants understand the difference in the psychological contract that operates in a participant-focussed learning environment. This psychological contract requires the learners to take on part of the responsibility for their own learning, with the help of the coach, to identify they ways in which they learn most effectively. These ways are not likely to be fixed and could change as learners gain confidence in managing. For example, it is not unusual for beginners to claim that they learn best by being told what to do. As they gain experience in learning in different ways, they begin to identify what works best.

Good coaching is about establishing a learning partnership with each group of participants.

Minimally, the participants should have the confidence to say the following to the coach, in a non-threatening manner:

- I don't understand what I'm being asked to do?
- What is the purpose of this exercise?
- I don't feel comfortable when you speak to me in that manner.
- Can you explain that in a different way rather than just repeating the instruction?
- Can we discuss how the class is organised?
- Can we talk about the objectives you want us to achieve?

Participants do not develop this confidence unless the coach actively creates and encourages an environment in which such questions can be asked and responded to in an open and positive manner. One way of setting an initial pattern is to consider discussing and agreeing on the principles by which the class will operate. An example is provided below.

- To develop competence in the use of the rowing machine so that the risk of strain of injury is reduced.
- To make the experience of developing as an indoor rower both challenging and fun.
- To support members in outlining routes/ options to develop and achieve their own goals within the sport.
- To establish an environment in which concerns can be discussed in an open and positive manner.
- To review these principles and the means by which they are being achieved.

There is a strong tendency for participants to blame themselves (rather than the coach) when they are feeling uncomfortable and, therefore, unable to make progress. 'I'm no good at this' is a common reaction. Your main objective as a coach should be to make participants feel good about themselves and what they have achieved as a result of your planning and inputs to the a session.

A BASIC CHECKLIST

In the first session did you:

- introduce yourself and outline your role?
- outline the broad aims and timetable for the session?
- check on any conditions that might limit what individuals could do (if not previously checked)?
- get to know the names of all of the participants?
- when talking to the whole group, arrange them so that you could eye contact everyone?
- when giving a demonstration, ensure that everyone was in a position to see clearly?
- quickly follow a demonstration with an opportunity to practise?
- use praise and encouragement to good effect?
- explain 'why' as well as 'what' and 'how'?
- succeed in establishing an environment in which participants asked questions?
- make the session both engaging and challenging?
- use a variety of methods to explain key points?
- use a variety of methods of closing the learning loop?
- provide a 'trailer' for the next session?
- thank participants for their contribution?
- identify what you would do next time to improve a similar session?

In sessions following did you, in addition:

- identify the three stages of development in your overall planning?
- change your session plan as a result of what did or did not happen in the preceding session?
- agree targets with individuals?
  celebrate successes?

Participants respond best to enthusiastic coaches – and are willing to ignore their other failings or limitations.

For further information on how to go about planning a coaching session, and all the tools you need to do this, including sample session plans and a self-assessment form, please refer to the Appendices (p. 164–172).

Summary
- Modern coaching styles are based on involving athletes in the process of improving their performance
- Good coaches have an understanding of the different ways in which people learn – and match their teaching to increase its effectiveness
- Good coaches regularly review their own performance based on feedback and how their athletes respond.

PHYSIOLOGY OF INDOOR ROWING

5

Competitive indoor rowing is one of the most physiologically demanding of all sporting activities. When competing in a standard 2000m indoor rowing race (lasting six to ten minutes), the metabolic rate of each competitor will increase by as much as twenty times normal resting metabolic rate. In order to support these high energy expenditures, indoor rowers must have excellent physiological abilities. In fact, the physiological demands of competitive indoor rowing are so great that success in national and international competitions is only possible after many months of dedicated training. On the other hand, there is no guarantee that a person who completes a substantial amount of training will experience substantial improvements in 2000m rowing performance. Significant gains in 2000m performance are only possible when a training program stimulates improvements in the key physiological systems.

For the competitive indoor rower seeking to make the best use of their training time, it is important to gain an understanding of the relationship between a person's physiological capabilities and their indoor rowing performance. Even for indoor rowers who are training for health rather than for performance, it is helpful to understand how the physiological systems of the body provide the energy for rowing training. Not only can this understanding serve to improve motivation, it can also enhance the ability of an indoor rower to make suitable modifications to their training. Such changes make it possible for an indoor rower to take control of their training and to make adjustments that can encourage superior gains in health and fitness.

UNDERSTANDING THE PHYSIOLOGY OF ROWING

Since 1980, scientists have published several hundred studies that examined the physiological demands of indoor rowing. Many of these studies are now freely accessible to interested readers and can be located using Google Scholar, PUBMED or other online research databases. Unfortunately, these studies are often complex, written in scientific jargon and the authors usually assume that the reader will have a good understanding of human physiology. In this chapter, we have attempted to report the findings of important scientific studies on indoor rowing and to do so with minimal technical detail. Important physiological terms are defined in various places to assist readers. Nevertheless, it is likely that some readers will still find sections of this chapter complex. It may be helpful to consult an introductory book on exercise physiology, such as *Sports Training Principles* by Dr Frank Dick.

DETERMINANTS OF INDOOR ROWING PERFORMANCE

Various features of an indoor rower can influence their 2000m performance ability. These features can usually be separated into one of the following performance-related categories:

- The psychological features of a rower (e.g. resilience; dedication; focus; motivation)
- The technique of a rower (e.g. body posture; coordination between legs, body and arms; stroke length)
- The physiological features of a rower (e.g. height; aerobic fitness; muscle strength and power).

Researchers have investigated the details of each performance category and this information has been helpful in explaining the separate and combined features of a rower that contribute to performance. As a result, much of what is required to achieve world-class indoor rowing performance is now understood.

In this chapter, we will focus on the physiology of indoor rowing and investigate the physiological features that contribute to successful 2000m indoor rowing performance. First, it is essential to understand that all three performance-related categories are closely interlinked. You only have to spend a little time near the rowing machines in a local gym to see evidence for this. Consider the tall, toned and physically impressive man who sits

down on a rowing machine next to another man half the size but who happens to be an experienced indoor rower. Despite the apparent physiological differences in size and muscle mass, it is the smaller individual who often outperforms the larger individual. In this example, the larger rower has not yet developed enough technical ability to make good use of his physiological advantages. Instead, the smaller man makes better combined use of his physiology and rowing technique to overcome the initial disadvantage.

Similar examples could be provided to show the importance of the psychological features of an indoor rower. Understanding the contribution of each specific factor believed to contribute to 2000m performance first requires an appreciation of the interaction between the psychological, physiological and technical abilities of a rower. This essential point must be kept in mind when reading the following sections that concentrate solely on the physiological features of a rower that determine indoor rowing performance.

WHAT ARE THE BENEFITS FROM A BETTER UNDERSTANDING OF THE PHYSIOLOGY OF INDOOR ROWING?

More than any other category, the physiology of successful indoor rowing performers has received the greatest amount of scientific investigation. The results of these investigations make it possible to isolate which physiological features are important to indoor rowing performance. This makes it easier to develop more effective methods of training and to understand what type of training will be effective and also helps to explain the benefits of nutrition, injury prevention strategies and new training devices.

There is good evidence to suggest that a specific set of physiological features can help explain the performance of indoor rowers. Indeed, it is possible to predict the 2000m race times of experienced indoor rowers to within 5 seconds using only a small selection of physiological measurements. This chapter presents a brief discussion of the physiological features of a rower that are important to 2000m indoor rowing performance. Where relevant, the effects of training on key physiological features are also described.

ENERGY DELIVERY DURING A 2000M COMPETITION

Before describing the relationship between 2000m performance and the physiological features of indoor rowers, it is first necessary to understand the importance of energy availability during rowing. The total amount of energy needed to complete a 2000m race is typically between 120 and 200kcal. This is roughly the amount of energy contained within one large banana and is a very small amount in comparison to the complete energy stores of a typical 75kg adult (50,000 to 100,000kcal). Under normal circumstances, 2000m indoor rowing performance is not limited by energy stores, but is instead restricted by the rate at which the energy is made available to the rower. In other words, there is still plenty of energy in the muscles of a rower after a 2000m race, but biochemical changes in the body (e.g. increasing muscle acidity) make it more difficult to use these energy stores.

Ultimately, all energy produced by the body depends on the availability of oxygen and the best

scientific estimates indicate that the aerobic system provides approximately 65 to 80 per cent of the energy need during a 2000m indoor rowing race. The anaerobic system supplies the remaining 20 to 35 per cent of the total energy requirement. Top indoor rowers will possess excellent abilities to sustain high rates of energy delivery from both the aerobic and anaerobic systems. In fact, the very best indoor rowers have recorded aerobic abilities that are among the highest values ever recorded for humans.

> The **aerobic system** refers to the chemical pathways that use oxygen to support energy production from stored fat and carbo-hydrate. It provides most of the energy for exercise tasks that last two or more minutes. Moderate or high intensity exercise, when performed for ten minutes or more, is usually suitable for improving the aerobic system.
>
> The **anaerobic system** refers to chemical pathways that can support energy production without the need for an immediate supply of oxygen. It provides most of the energy for exercise tasks of maximal or near maximal intensity when performed for less than two minutes.

THE PHYSIOLOGICAL REQUIREMENTS OF TOP INDOOR ROWERS

This section presents information about the specific physiological features that are important for rowing performance.

The following physiological features are required to be a top rower:

- Above average height (open class competitors only)
- High absolute aerobic power (VO_2max; >4 litres per minute for open women and >5.5 litres per minute for open men
- The ability to sustain 95–100 per cent of maximum aerobic power for 2000m
- A high lactate threshold
- A fast responding oxygen delivery system at the onset of a 2000m race
- A high ventilation capacity
- A breathing pattern that is well-synchronised to the different phases of the rowing stroke
- A high anaerobic peak power and capacity
- High strength levels, especially when measured at medium movement speeds
- A well-developed ability to resist muscular fatigue (including acid buffering capacity)
- High power output to body weight ratio
- Low relative body fat; ≤12 per cent for open men and ≤20 per cent for women
- High fat-free mass content
- A high mechanical efficiency.

HEIGHT

Most people think that the best rowers are usually tall in stature. Indeed, the top open weight indoor rowers are typically taller than the average person. It is also highly unlikely that a diminutive man or women will ever threaten the official 2000m indoor rowing world records for open men or women. On the other hand, top lightweight competitors are usually of normal height. When the heights of large numbers of indoor rowers are compared to 2000m performance, the correlations are typically low to moderate at best.

So why do tall open weight rowers appear to have more success than shorter open weight rowers? The usual explanation is that greater height increases effective stroke length. Direct measurements obtained during indoor rowing racing have confirmed that, on average, tall rowers exhibit longer stroke lengths than shorter rowers. But the actual gain in average stroke length can be small and is often less than 10cm between rowers who can differ in height by as much as 30cm. It's possible that height is a better indirect predictor of rowing performance than a direct predictor. Since other important features, including weight and aerobic power, are known to increase with standing height, it may be that the small advantage enjoyed by tall open weight competitors is only indirectly related to height. Also, the often substantial improvements in 2000m performance following a period of training clearly are not linked to height since this will be the same before and after training. In summary, a person's height is probably of minor importance to indoor rowing performance and certainly of less importance than popular opinion would suggest.

BODY WEIGHT

A large body weight is another feature that is often thought to be important for rowing performance. Competition results from the Concept2 indoor race series, along with a number of scientific studies, show that body weight correlates well with performance. The body weights of top indoor rowing competitors in the open weight category are usually between 90 and 100kg for men and between 70 and 80kg for women. By comparison, the average weight of untrained individuals of similar age (20 to 30 years) living in Western countries such as Australia, the United Kingdom and the United States is typically between 75 and 80kg for men and between 57 and 62kg for women.

Body weight has an important effect on the energy cost of various physical activities. For example, runners have to spend a large proportion of total energy availability supporting the movement of their full body weight. Indoor rowers direct a lower proportion of total energy to meet to the energy cost of body movement, in part because indoor rowing requires very little work against gravity. If a 5kg weight was strapped to the waist of a 75kg runner, it would substantially increase the difficulty and energy cost. However, if this procedure was repeated during rowing, the increase in difficulty would be much less. Indoor rowers still have to use much of their energy to move the body and this becomes more obvious as stroke rates increase. Approximately 35 per cent of the energy cost of rowing at 32 strokes per minute is due to body movement. In other words, a large amount of the energy produced by the body during rowing does not contribute to the power output recorded on the computer display. The energy cost of body movement increases in proportion to stroke rate and the body weight of the rower.

Based on the average 2000m performances of top indoor rowers, lightweight competitors record times that are usually 5–6 per cent slower than open weight competitors within the same age and sex divisions. This equates to a 1 per cent improvement in 2000m performance for every 4kg of additional body weight. It is also noteworthy that relatively few open weight competitors record 2000m performances faster than 6 minutes for men and 7 minutes for women, yet the current world records for both lightweight men and women are both slightly quicker than these critical times. Nevertheless, the world records for open weight men and women are still between 20 and 30 seconds faster than for lightweight competitors. Body weight is clearly associated with 2000m performance, but similar to the observations made for height and rowing performance, the reasons why heavier individuals outperform lighter individuals requires further explanation. In particular, body composition is a critical factor to consider when evaluating the relationship between 2000m indoor rowing performance and body weight.

Measuring body composition

The human body consists of various chemicals, fluids, minerals and tissues. The diverse distribution of these components throughout the body makes it hard to obtain precise measures of total body composition. However, it is much easier to obtain reasonable estimates of total body fat using affordable measurement techniques such as skinfold analysis or bioelectrical impedance (bathroom weight scales often use this method) as well as more accurate measures such as DXA scanning (which uses two X-ray beams of different energy) or air and water displacement techniques. Once total body fat is known, everything else in the body is considered the fat free mass. The major component of fat free mass is lean muscle tissue. Regular indoor rowing can increase total fat free mass and decrease total fat mass.

RELATIVE BODY FAT OF INDOOR ROWERS

Research suggests that the relative body fat of top indoor rowers is similar to that of other endurance athletes. Successful open weight competitors will normally have relative body fats that range from 8 to 12 per cent for men and from 15 to 20 per cent for women. These values are lower than would be expected in untrained individuals of similar body size. A healthy young man would normally have a relative body fat of about 15 per cent, while a healthy young woman would normally be around 25 per cent. Predictably, lightweight indoor rowers usually have far less body fat than both untrained individuals and open weight rowers, with lightweight men typically between 5 and 10 per cent and lightweight women between 12 and 18 per cent. Although, genes do influence a person's relative body fat, it is the dietary habits and training strategies of successful indoor rowers that better explain their lower body fat.

> Fat mass consists of all body weight that is fat tissue and includes the fat contents located in the interior of bones, muscles and organs. Fat free mass consists of all other body weight that is not fat tissue.

FAT FREE MASS OF INDOOR ROWERS

2000m indoor rowing performance is strongly correlated with a rower's total fat free mass, whereas total fat mass is a relatively poor predictor of performance. In fact, the observation that heavier rowers tend to outperform lighter rowers is mostly due to differences in fat free mass favouring heavier rowers. The fat mass of a rower does not contribute to power output during rowing and any additional fat mass is acting as dead weight to increase the energy cost of movement.

When the independent effects of fat mass and fat free mass on rowing performance are understood, then the importance of body weight to performance can be better appreciated. Heavier rowers typically outperform lighter rowers due to their greater amounts of fat free mass, and although heavier rowers are also likely to have higher amounts of fat mass, there is much more benefit to having higher amounts of fat free mass than there is penalty for having higher amounts of fat mass. In cases where lighter rowers outperform heavier rowers it is worth considering to what extent such differences are due to higher amounts of fat free mass in the lighter rower even though overall body weight may be lower.

Changes in both fat mass and fat free mass after several months of regular training make important contributions to changes in indoor rowing performance. These changes in body composition are often not detected by indoor rowers. When a person begins regular indoor rowing, they may expect to lose body weight soon after. However, the extra calories expended through training are often replaced by a proportional increase in food intake with the result that body weight does not change. But, body composition often improves even in the absence of overall weight change since indoor rowing can increase fat free mass in the rowing muscles. Also, the fat mass stores in the hips, thighs and stomach typically decrease in size and while most of this fat will leave the body, some of it will actually end up being stored deep inside the rowing muscles and used to fuel training. In fact, the combination of greater fat stores and increased amounts of aerobic enzymes inside the rowing muscles explains much of the improvement in endurance capacity from training. For these reasons, it is recommended that indoor rowers track their changes in body composition and not just body weight, especially during the first six to twelve months of training when changes in fat mass and fat free mass are often greatest.

VENTILATION AND BREATHING PATTERN

The ventilation system of indoor rowers must be capable of providing high volumes of air to deliver oxygen to the blood. In order to achieve internationally competitive performances in the open category, men must be capable of inspiring at least 200 litres of air each minute and women must be able to inspire in excess of 140 litres of air each minute. These values are approximately twice the expected levels for untrained individuals (matched for age and body size) and develop in response to indoor rowing training and a strengthening of the respiratory muscles. Improved breathing patterns may also help explain the improved capabilities of top rowers. In contrast, the physical size of an indoor rower's lungs is unchanged by regular rowing training.

The amount of air delivered to the lungs during rowing is directly proportional to the intensity of exercise and is the product of the number of breaths per minute (breathing rate) and amount of air inspired per breath (tidal volume).

Ventilation changes during rowing are closely related to the oxygen demand of exercise and are tightly controlled by the amount of carbon dioxide released by the active muscles.

- When the pace of rowing increases, the active muscles release more carbon dioxide into the blood which stimulates an increase in ventilation.
- Initially, the increase in ventilation is achieved through increases in tidal volume. When exercise becomes more intense, tidal volume eventually cannot increase further and breathing frequency increases.
- Tidal volume and breathing frequency may be affected by the unique task demands of indoor rowing.

Scientists at Dartmouth Medical School in the United States measured the breathing patterns of experienced rowers as well as non-rowers during indoor rowing on a Concept2 machine. The specific point in the stroke cycle when each subject began to inhale was recorded, both during sub-maximal and maximal rowing. The non-rowers were unable to connect their breathing to the separate phases of the stroke and simply breathed at random. Experienced rowers, on the other hand, clearly synchronised their breathing to match the different phases of the rowing stroke. When rowing at 18 strokes per minute (sub-maximal), experienced rowers required one complete breath per stroke and typically began to inhale at the start of the recovery phase, expiring during the drive phase. When rowing at maximal effort (2000m race pace), experienced rowers completed two breaths per stroke. Breathing patterns remained well matched to stroke phases, inhaling once at the beginning of the recovery phase and then again around the catch phase. Expirations occurred during both the recovery and drive phases. In a separate study, the same researchers reported that novice rowers develop these consistent breathing patterns after several months of rowing training, without any need for specific coaching.

German researchers confirmed the use of the distinct two breaths per stroke pattern in experienced rowers during high intensity rowing. They also found important differences between the size of the two breaths. A greater volume of air was inspired during the breath taken in the early recovery than the breath taken at the catch. This suggests that there may be physical limits to breathing during high intensity indoor rowing due to the compressed position of the upper body at the catch. Additionally, the muscles that normally assist deep inspiration are also important for stabilising the upper body. Upper body stability is essential to the production of high power output during the drive phase of maximal intensity rowing, making it more difficult for a rower to inhale during this phase of the stroke. These restrictions to breathing during intense rowing may result in small but important reductions in the uptake of oxygen via the lungs. This possibility is more likely to occur in top indoor rowers due to the extremely high ventilation rates achieved by these athletes. There are also suggestions that respiratory muscles may develop fatigue during intense indoor rowing. Given these different possible restrictions on breathing during indoor rowing, it may be possible to improve rowing performance by targeting specific ways to improve breathing during rowing.

Improving the strength of respiratory muscles has been suggested to improve indoor rowing performance. Researchers at Birmingham University in England invited 14 competitive female rowers to add respiratory muscle training to their normal rowing activities for 11 weeks. All rowers completed 60 deep breaths each day using a Powerbreathe device that restricts air flow during each breath and provides a form of overload to the respiratory muscles. Half the rowers performed maximal inspirations against a resistance of 50 per cent of their peak inspiratory capacity (experimental group) while the other half performed maximal inspirations against a resistance of only 15 per cent of their peak inspiratory capacity (control group). The maximal inspiratory pressure (measured at rest) achieved by the experimental group increased by 45 per cent, but was unchanged in the control group. The time to complete a 5000m test, performed before and after the 11 weeks, improved by 36 seconds in the experimental group (+3.1 per cent) compared with only 11 seconds improvement in the control group (+0.9 per cent). The researchers suggested that the performance enhancing effects from using inspiratory muscle training may have been due to a reduction in respiratory muscle fatigue during rowing. Inspiratory muscle training might also improve the volume of air inspired during the shorter breath that typically occurs at the catch, possibly improving the efficiency of breathing.

Powerbreathe devices (see figure 5.1) are now popular with indoor rowers and the results described above provide some support for their use. However, there is still much uncertainty about the benefits of inspiratory muscle training. Also, the conclusions of the Birmingham study may have been affected by the lower inspiratory abilities of the experimental group at baseline compared to the control group. This difference may have improved the prospects for increasing inspiratory strength and rowing performance in the experimental group. Future studies are necessary to confirm if respiratory muscle training really does improve indoor rowing performance.

Table 5.1	Respiratory muscle training and 5000m ergometer rowing performance		
Group	Powerbreathe resistance used during respiratory training sessions	Improvement over 5000m	Percentage improvement
Experimental group	50% of peak inspiratory capacity	36s	3.1%
Control group	15% of peak inspiratory capacity	11s	0.9%

Source: Data from Volianitis, S. et al. (2001)

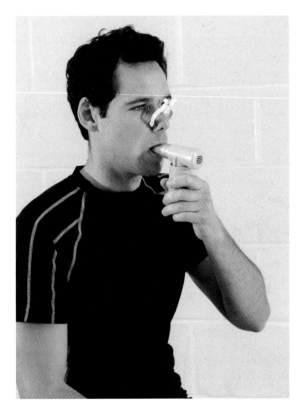

Fig 5.1 Powerbreathe device

LACTATE THRESHOLD

Endurance athletes often talk about the importance of training to developing a high lactate threshold to improve performance. During exercise, the active muscles can increase the rate of energy supplied from glucose metabolism by producing lactic acid through the process of anaerobic glycolysis. As soon as the lactic acid is formed, however, it is rapidly converted to lactate after releasing a hydrogen ion. The formed lactate is then released from the muscle and can be measured in the blood of the exercising person. The lactate will be used elsewhere in the body, usually as an energy source. By measuring the blood lactate concentration, it is possible to make inferences about the acidity levels inside active muscles and to use this information to make accurate predictions about the endurance performance capabilities of an athlete. The term 'lactate threshold' specifically refers to the exercise intensity at which blood lactate levels begin to increase above baseline (see figure 5.2).

There is a range of terminology in current use to describe the same basic change in blood lactate concentration during exercise. These include lactate turnpoint, anaerobic threshold and ventilatory threshold. The reasons why some scientists prefer to use these terms are not important for the present discussion and we will continue to use the term lactate threshold. What is important to note is that the lactate threshold of an indoor rower is both an excellent predictor

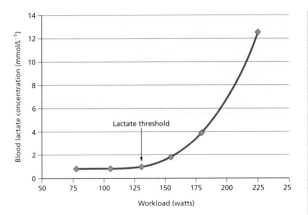

Fig 5.2 Measurement of the blood lactate threshold during indoor rowing

Lactate threshold refers to exercise intensity where the concentration of lactate in the blood increases above baseline levels. It is very sensitive to training status and is frequently used by sport scientists to help show if physiological improvements have occurred. Lactate threshold information can also help establish suitable intensities for training.

of 2000m performance and a useful measure for tracking the improvements from endurance training.

Lactate threshold is very sensitive to the training status of an indoor rower. As the volume or intensity of rowing training increases, the amount of mitochondria and the concentration of aerobic enzymes inside the rowing muscles also increase. The mitochondria are the powerhouses of the muscle which contain the essential biological machinery and aerobic enzymes necessary to extract energy from stored fat and carbohydrate. Oxygen must also be available in order to support this transfer of chemical energy. The significance of these intramuscular changes is that they allow the rower to increase the rate of aerobic energy production and to increase the rower's ability to use either fat or carbohydrate as a fuel source for energy production. Coaches often use lactate threshold data to prescribe appropriate training intensities for an indoor rower. Lactate threshold is highly correlated with the maximal aerobic power of a rower.

AEROBIC AND ANAEROBIC POWER
Aerobic power

During a 2000m race, competitive rowers reach their limit for aerobic energy production within the first few minutes (see figure 5.3). This limit is termed maximal aerobic power or abbreviated to its scientific name, VO_2max. Various physiological factors influence VO_2max including body size, fat free mass, number and size of mitochondria, heart size and blood volume. VO_2max is also influenced by an indoor rower's training status, sex and age. Scientists generally agree that the major factor that limits oxygen use during exercise is the available supply of oxygen to the active muscles rather than any limitation to use oxygen within the muscles.

A high VO_2max value is an essential prerequisite for anyone who wants to compete successfully at the international level. In fact, the very best openweight indoor rowers in the world have recorded VO_2max values that are some of the highest ever achieved by humans! Typically, a woman needs to possess a VO_2max in excess of 4.5 litres per minute to row 2000m in a time of 6 minutes 40 seconds, while a man will require a VO_2max of at least 5.5 litres per minute to break

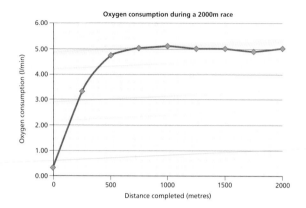

Fig 5.3 Oxygen consumption during a 2000m ergometer race

For a direct assessment of VO_2max, the test should normally be performed on a rowing machine, although a treadmill or cycle ergometer can be used. The rower must wear a mouthpiece or facemask that directs all of the expired air into a gas collection system for analysis of total air volume as well as oxygen and carbon dioxide concentrations. The test usually lasts between 10 and 30 minutes and involves rowing at progressively faster work rates until further increases in work are no longer possible. The VO_2max of the rower is likely to occur during the final few minutes of the test and is reported based on the highest volume of oxygen that was extracted from the atmosphere during a single minute.

the 6 minute barrier. These rates of oxygen use are approximately double the normal values for healthy young men and women.

It is possible to estimate 2000m race time if VO_2max is known or vice versa. Several websites offer online calculators that provide a reasonable estimate of VO_2max from a known 2000m race time (e.g. http://www.concept2.com/). Specialist test facilities, including equipment to measure the amount of oxygen removed from the atmosphere, are needed to obtain a true measure of VO_2max.

Most universities will have a sport science department where VO_2max is routinely measured and it is often possible to arrange an individual test (see figure 5.4). Fitness professionals sometimes offer VO_2max measurements for a fee, but these are usually indirect tests where VO_2max is estimated from heart rate and don't involve direct measurements of oxygen use. These indirect estimates, while useful and interesting, are unlikely to exceed the accuracy of estimates obtained using a recent 2000m time.

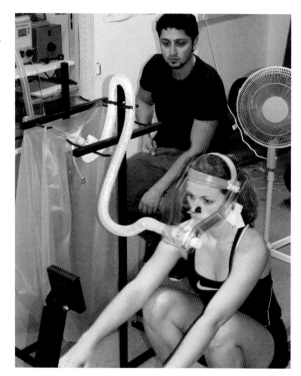

Fig 5.4 Measurement of VO_2max with an indoor rower

While 2000m rowing performance is highly correlated with the amount of oxygen that an indoor rower uses in one minute, it is also important to be able to sustain a high rate of oxygen use for as long as possible. Most indoor rowers will reach 95–100 per cent of their VO_2max during the first 2 minutes of a race and remain near this level for the remainder of the race. The average per cent of VO_2max sustained during indoor competition is reasonably similar between indoor rowers, even when there are relatively large differences in performance times. However, there will still be predictable differences in the volumes of oxygen used by each rower, but these are almost entirely due to the existing differences in VO_2max. Accordingly, training strategies that enhance VO_2max are likely to provide the greatest benefits to 2000m indoor rowing performance.

Effects of training on aerobic power

Scientific research has revealed that while endurance training can substantially increase the VO_2max of most people, the effects of training vary greatly from person to person. Studies that have measured groups of untrained individuals before and after a 20 week standardised endurance training programme show typical improvements in VO_2max of approximately 20 per cent. The physiological changes that are responsible for the increase in VO_2max are also primarily responsible for the associated improvements in endurance capacity. Interestingly, some untrained individuals enjoy large gains in VO_2max from a standard aerobic training programme, improving by as much as 50 per cent of the starting VO_2max. On the other hand, some untrained individuals hardly increase VO_2max at all despite adhering to the same well-designed endurance training plans.

However, it is still possible to increase endurance capacity and gain large health benefits from exercise even if VO_2max doesn't change. Likewise, 2000m indoor rowing performance can still improve even without an increase in VO_2max, but the size of the improvement is usually small.

By studying the endurance training responses of families as well as identical and non-identical twins, scientists have estimated that approximately 50 per cent of a person's ability to improve VO_2max with aerobic training is influenced by their genes. Adhering to an appropriate training programme is critical to developing a high VO_2max, but ultimately a person's genetic inheritance will set the upper limit to possible improvements in VO_2max, which then imposes the main limit to their 2000m indoor rowing performance.

Having established that most of the difference in 2000m performance between trained rowers is explained by differences in oxygen use, it is worth considering what other physiological features limit indoor rowing performance. Indeed, rowers who possess identical VO_2max values can still differ in true 2000m race performance by as much as 10 seconds. These marginal differences in time are still important in determining final competitive placing during indoor races. Although non-physiological factors such as psychological drive will help explain some of these small performance differences, the effects of anaerobic capability and mechanical efficiency are important physiological considerations.

Anaerobic power

The rate of energy production supplied by the ATP phosphocreatine and anaerobic glycolytic systems is termed anaerobic power. Athletes who compete in brief, high intensity sporting events such as weightlifting and 100m sprinting have extremely high abilities to supply anaerobic power. Successful athletes in these events typically possess high levels of fat free mass and a high proportion of fast twitch muscle fibres in the muscle groups that are of primary importance in the particular sporting event. These fibres also contain very high concentrations of key anaerobic enzymes. It is interesting to note that the VO_2max values of top competitors in predominantly anaerobic events are reasonably similar to the values of healthy but non-aerobically trained individuals.

ATP molecules are packets of chemical energy. Muscles can only use energy when it is in the form of ATP. Ultimately, all of the energy that is used to power muscle contractions comes from ATP produced by the aerobic and anaerobic systems.

At present, there is no way to measure the true anaerobic capabilities of an athlete with a high degree of accuracy. Instead, the anaerobic systems of rowers are indirectly assessed using sprint and explosive power assessments where better performances are assumed to reflect superior anaerobic power. One popular test of anaerobic power is the 30 second sprint test using the indoor rowing machine. This test actually attempts to measure both the maximal anaerobic power as well as the capacity of the rower to maintain high rates of anaerobic power. Maximal anaerobic power is recorded as the highest power output obtained during one stroke and this usually occurs in the first five strokes. Anaerobic capacity is recorded as the average power for the full 30 second effort. One major problem that occurs when anaerobic capacity measurements are made using a 30 second sprint is that some of the ATP used during this test will be produced by the aerobic rather than the anaerobic system. The anaerobic system is the exclusive source of the ATP for the first six seconds of a sprint. Thereafter, the aerobic system starts to provide some of the ATP which contributes to 30 second sprint performance. This means that an athlete's performance in the 30 second anaerobic capacity test will also be influenced by their aerobic system. At present, there is no test method that can accurately identify an athlete's true anaerobic capacity.

When used in isolation, anaerobic power tests are not especially helpful to predicting 2000m performance. In groups of trained rowers, the athletes who record the highest anaerobic scores are rarely the same athletes who record the fastest 2000m times. However, the ability to accurately predict 2000m indoor race times is slightly improved when anaerobic test scores are combined with aerobic test scores. In other words, the anaerobic test scores of two indoor rowers who have identical VO_2max scores may help explain differences in their 2000m performances.

Balance between aerobic and anaerobic power

Indoor rowers ideally require high levels of both aerobic and anaerobic power. As mentioned earlier, the maximal aerobic power recorded by top indoor rowers are among the best scores of any athlete. However, the maximal anaerobic power scores recorded for top indoor rowers, while impressive in comparison to normal adults, are still well below the scores of top weightlifters and sprint athletes. In theory, a world-class indoor rower should be able to gain significant additional advantage from increasing their maximal anaerobic power to a similar level to that of top weightlifters and sprinters. In practice, there appears to be a significant amount of interference between the physiological adaptations needed to achieve extreme values for maximal anaerobic and maximal aerobic power. The interference phenomenon helps explain why gains in maximal anaerobic power following weeks of anaerobic conditioning work are reduced when significant amounts of aerobic training are included in the training programme. Despite the important contribution from anaerobic power during 2000m indoor rowing, it appears that the conditioning practices of top indoor rowers place greater emphasis on the development of aerobic power.

While strength and conditioning experts and researchers are currently investigating ways to minimise or even eliminate the interference between these two systems of energy production, at present, it is the aerobic capabilities of the athlete that best predict 2000m performance. If high status indoor rowing events such as the European or World Championships offered a sprint category (e.g.100m), then it is reasonable to expect that the physiological capabilities of the 100m winner would be considerably different from the winner of the equivalent class over the 2000m distance. The best indoor sprint rowers would probably have significantly higher maximal anaerobic power but lower maximal aerobic power in comparison with the best 2000m indoor rowers. These physiological differences would partly reflect differences in training approaches. Sprint rowers would almost

certainly log far less kilometres of indoor rowing each year and this rowing would be at a much higher average intensity than the traditional approach used by 2000m rowers. Sprint rowers would also dedicate larger amounts of training time to weightlifting with the goal of increasing total fat free mass to levels well above the values typically observed for top 2000m indoor rowers.

Training for optimal levels of anaerobic power

A comprehensive training plan for indoor rowing must address the need to develop optimal levels of anaerobic power. The concept of optimal anaerobic power is distinct from that of maximal anaerobic power and involves training to achieve the greatest possible increase in anaerobic power without significantly compromising either aerobic power or 2000m performance. Anaerobic power is best developed through the use of specific and non-specific resistance training methods. Specific resistance training can be performed on the indoor rowing machine with high drag factors (resistance control set to the heaviest/hardest positions). Non-specific resistance training usually involves traditional weightlifting exercises in a gym and can produce substantial gains in fat free mass after eight weeks. For large gains in fat free mass to occur, energy intake should also be increased though the addition of between 500 and 750kcal to a standard diet.

It is important to understand that anaerobic power can increase even when there are no alterations to body composition or improvements in fat free mass. For example, an athlete's ability to produce maximal force will increase if the brain allows more of the available muscle fibres to be recruited during a maximal effort. Under normal circumstances, the brain will protect the muscles from damage by limiting the number of muscle fibres that contract. While it may seem strange that the brain deliberately prevents all of the muscle fibres from contracting during a maximal effort, it does so to prevent muscle damage and to avoid tearing the muscle from the connection points on the bones (tendons). It is likely that resistance training improves neuromuscular activity and enhances force production by allowing more of the available muscle mass to contribute to the movement.

MECHANICAL EFFICIENCY DURING INDOOR ROWING

Each rower's capability to achieve a high rate of energy production during a 2000m race will be an important influence on his or her actual performance. This rate reflects the combined output of the aerobic and anaerobic systems and represents the ultimate limit to 2000m rowing performance. However, the actual power output achieved during indoor rowing is determined by each person's ability to convert the available aerobic and anaerobic energy into useful mechanical output (e.g. flywheel revolutions per minute). The ratio of power production relative to the total energy supply is called 'mechanical efficiency'.

Physiologists can measure mechanical efficiency during rowing by expressing power output as a percentage of the energy expenditure of the rower. Power output is displayed on the performance monitor of the rowing machine and energy expenditure is usually recorded from measurements of oxygen consumption and carbon dioxide production. Physiologists sometimes express rowing power or speed relative to the rate of oxygen consumption, eliminating the need for additional information to calculate actual energy expenditure. This measurement is called 'economy' and is sometimes used by exercise physiologists as an alternative to calculating mechanical efficiency.

Unfortunately, it is currently not possible to obtain a true measurement of mechanical efficiency during a 2000m race because of the difficulties involved in measuring anaerobic energy production during maximum efforts. For this reason, the mechanical efficiency or economy of a rower is typically measured at exercise intensities below the lactate threshold, where the contribution from anaerobic energy sources is usually considered to be negligible. This methodological problem makes it much harder to explain the true importance of mechanical efficiency to indoor rowing performance and should be kept in mind when reading the following information.

Mechanical efficiency and indoor rowing performance

The mechanical efficiency of indoor rowers is likely to be an important determinant of 2000m performance. But few researchers have investigated this possibility despite the obvious theoretical importance. Measurements of mechanical efficiency during moderate intensity indoor rowing typically reveal values that range from 15 to 25 per cent depending on how researchers control for confounding effects such as stroke rate, flywheel resistance and the basal metabolic rates of rowers. In other words, only a small proportion of a rower's energy is converted to useful mechanical power. Instead, most of the energy produced during rowing is used to generate heat and is easily detected by the rower. Under normal circumstances, this heat contributes to the increase in body temperature and stimulates sweat production. Accordingly, high efficiency rowers (i.e. mechanical efficiency values of >20 per cent) should be better equipped to cope with hot environmental conditions due to lower rates of heat production. These benefits will be of greatest importance during long training sessions or competitions lasting 30 minutes or more.

> Basal metabolic rate refers to the minimum energy requirement needed to maintain the vital organs of the body. If a person gains additional muscle through resistance training, then basal metabolic rate will increase to support the extra demand for energy from the extra muscle mass.

To date, the best evidence to support the theoretical link between mechanical efficiency and 2000m rowing performance is provided by a laboratory-based study of top French oarsmen. Researchers from Lyon University measured the submaximal mechanical efficiency of 54 elite lightweight and heavyweight oarsmen while rowing on a Concept2 ergometer. The mechanical efficiency of each rower was correlated with their 2000m ergometer performance. This study is particularly noteworthy because of the large numbers of subjects studied, as well as the impressive 2000m times of all subjects. Specifically, average 2000m time was 6 minutes 5 seconds for the heavyweight rowers (n=31; where 'n' represents the number of subjects) and 6 minutes 21 seconds for the lightweight rowers (n=23). Average mechanical efficiency was 18.5 per cent with a range of values between 15 and 22 per cent. There was no difference in the average efficiency of lightweight and heavyweight rowers.

Overall, the mechanical efficiency of each rower accounted for 12 per cent of the variation in 2000m performance time. However, when these results were re-analysed after separating the oarsmen by weight classification, mechanical efficiency became a better predictor, accounting for 26 per cent and 41 per cent of the variation in 2000m performance for lightweight and heavyweight oarsmen, respectively. This research suggests that mechanical efficiency may start to emerge as an important determinant of 2000m indoor rowing performance when the influence of size-dependent performance factors (e.g. absolute VO_2max and fat free mass) are reduced by making comparisons between well-trained rowers of a similar size.

Does an indoor rower's physiology affect their mechanical efficiency during rowing?

If mechanical efficiency is confirmed as an important determinant of 2000m indoor rowing performance, then it would be especially interesting to learn why some indoor rowers have high efficiencies while others have comparatively low efficiencies. It would also be helpful to know if efficiency changes with indoor rowing training so that improved training methods could be developed to specifically enhance mechanical efficiency. There is some evidence that cyclists can improve their mechanical efficiency after many years of cycling training by as much as 20 per cent (i.e. increasing from a measured value of 15 per cent to 18 per cent). These improvements in efficiency may be due to changes in muscle fibre recruitment patterns which allow the energy cost of cycling to be more evenly distributed across the available muscle mass, reducing the metabolic stress on each muscle fibre. Interestingly, cyclists who possess high mechanical efficiency also have greater proportions of slow twitch muscle fibres in their leg muscles. Potentially, large amounts of cycling training may promote favourable changes in slow twitch muscle fibre activity which may enhance overall mechanical efficiency during cycling. On the other hand, it may be that muscle fibre composition per se is the major determinant of mechanical efficiency during exercise. If so, then the high mechanical efficiency of some indoor rowers may be due to greater proportions of slow twitch fibres in the primary rowing muscles.

Muscle fibre type is largely determined by a person's genes, as revealed in studies of identical twins who are found to have near identical proportions of slow and fast twitch fibres. Nevertheless, growing evidence suggests that endurance training can result in small increases in the proportion of slow twitch fibres (up to 10 per cent change) and it is clearly the case that the size of each muscle fibre can be substantially altered through training. Therefore, while both the size and proportion of slow twitch fibres in initially untrained identical twins will be similar, if one twin performs regular endurance training, significant differences in these physiological features can develop. In this way, genetic factors are understood to make an important contribution to indoor rowing performance, but greater importance should be attached to the interaction

between a person's genes and other critical features such as the amount and type of training performed, the diet of the rower and the extent to which rowing skill has been developed.

Olympic rowers usually have higher proportions of slow twitch muscle fibres than a normal adult, although considerable individual variability exists. Slow twitch fibres account for approximately 70 per cent of the total fibre population in the leg muscles of a typical Olympic rower. However, some Olympic rowers have about 50 per cent slow twitch fibres, a value which is similar to that found in untrained individuals. If muscle fibre type is found to be an important determinant of mechanical efficiency during indoor rowing, then these basic differences in fibre proportions could help explain why some experienced indoor rowers may have lower mechanical efficiency than comparatively inexperienced rowers. However, extensive research provided by Dr Fritz Hagerman of Ohio University suggests that muscle fibre composition does not change in response to rowing training.

Dr Hagerman has measured the physiological responses of candidates for the American national team for over 30 years. His research supports the idea that mechanical efficiency may improve with rowing training. For example, several athletes improved their 2000m ergometer performance over a period of eight years, yet their rate of oxygen consumption during the 2000m test did not improve. Possible explanations for these results include improvements in mechanical efficiency during rowing, increases in anaerobic power or a combination of both. Dr Hagerman suggested that improvements in rowing technique, rather than changes in the proportion of slow twitch muscle fibres (which were also measured), are more likely to explain the improvements in rowing efficiency after several years of training. However, it is unclear if these physiological based measurements of mechanical efficiency actually reflect the skill level of the rower. The next section of this chapter examines this issue in greater detail.

Do changes in indoor rowing technique alter mechanical efficiency?

Despite the previous suggestions that mechanical efficiency during indoor rowing may be influenced by the technique of a rower, there is limited support for this idea. Many rowers and coaches assume that stroke technique has a major influence in determining 2000m indoor rowing performance. The challenge, however, is to find clear evidence that stroke technique is linked to performance in groups of trained indoor rowers. For example, are there any consistent differences in technique between elite and intermediate indoor rowers? The results of several biomechanical investigations comparing stroke technique in elite and intermediate rowers show limited support for consistent differences between groups.

It is interesting to note that world class 2000m indoor rowing performances have been achieved by highly trained runners, swimmers and even rugby players within several months of beginning indoor rowing training. Potentially, it may be possible to achieve an efficient rowing technique after a short period of specific rowing training. Indeed, this was the conclusion of Australian researchers at Deakin University who recorded the physiological and technical changes of a group of young men during their first weeks of regular indoor rowing.

Dr Tony Sparrow and colleagues recruited six physically fit young men who had no background of regular indoor rowing. The men performed 10 sessions of rowing on a Concept2 ergometer at 100w for 16 minutes per session. At no time during the study did the men receive any technique instruction and were effectively free to select their own stroke technique. On average, the 10 sessions were completed within six weeks. Rowing economy improved by an average of 9 per cent between session 1 and session 10 and was accompanied by improvements in leg and arm muscle activity as well as stroke to stroke consistency (obtained using handle force profiles; see Chapter 8 for more details). Training reduced the perceived difficulty of rowing. There was also a tendency to increase stroke length but this did not reach the threshold for statistical significance. The researchers also noted that self-selected stroke rate decreased from an average of 28 strokes per minute (session 1) to 22 strokes per minute (session 10). There was no change in the VO_2max of the men before and after the training period (measured on a cycle ergometer), thus reducing the potential for the improved economy to be due to changes in aerobic fitness changes.

The exact reason(s) for the 9 per cent reduction in the oxygen cost of rowing (i.e. economy) are difficult to identify, but the use of slower stroke rates and increases in force production per stroke are likely explanations. Additionally, Sparrow and colleagues suggested that an improved synergy between muscle groups as well as a greater recruitment of individual muscle fibres within the primary rowing muscles may also have contributed to the enhancement of rowing economy. These interesting results suggest that rowing technique becomes increasingly stable and economical after only a brief period of initial training, even in the absence of formal instruction. They also demonstrate the potential for self-improvement in rowing technique which may correlate with improvements in rowing efficiency. Nevertheless, it would be unwise to extrapolate these results to groups of experienced indoor rowers. The differences in mechanical efficiency and economy values between top indoor rowers may simply reflect inherent physiological features such as muscle fibre composition. There may be very limited potential to make alterations to mechanical efficiency through training or technique changes. Hopefully, future research studies will provide a better understanding of the factors that determine mechanical efficiency.

PHYSIOLOGICAL DIFFERENCES ACROSS DIFFERENT LEVELS OF INDOOR ROWING PERFORMANCE

Additional data is presented in figure 5.5 to help clarify the extent to which differences in 2000m indoor rowing performance may be associated with annual training volumes and selected physiological parameters. The individual values are representative of the expected average values for each performance level and were estimated using the results of a large selection of research studies.

	Open Men (25 years of age)			Open Women (25 years of age)		
2000m time (min:sec)	8:00	7:00	6:00	8:45	7:45	6:45
100m sprint time (sec)	20:3	17:2	14:1	23:0	19:3	16:2
Years of indoor rowing training	1	3	5	1	3	5
Annual volume of indoor rowing (km)	1500	3000	4500	1250	2500	4700
Height (cm)	190	190	180	180	180	180
Body mass (kg)	90	90	90	75	75	75
Fat mass (kg)	18.0	13.5	9.0	18.8	15.0	11.3
Fat free mass (kg)	72.0	76.5	81.0	56.3	60.0	63.8
Body fat (% of body mass)	20	15	10	25	20	15
Maximum heart rate (beats/min)	187	187	187	190	190	190
Absolute VO_2max (l/min)	3.7	5.2	6.8	2.7	3.7	4.7
Relative VO_2max (ml/kg body mass/min)	41	58	75	36	49	63
Maximum ventilation (l/min)	120	168	220	87	120	152
Slow twitch muscle fibres (%)	55	65	75	55	65	75
Mechanical efficiency (%)	16	18	20	16	18	20

Fig 5.5 Comparison of selected physiological values in different indoor rowers

INDOOR ROWING TRAINING FOR HEALTH AND PERFORMANCE

6

Regular physical activity is widely understood to be an essential part of a healthy lifestyle. Nevertheless, large numbers of children and adults in western countries do very little physical activity and often live sedentary lifestyles. Yet, many of these sedentary and inactive people would not consider themselves so, particularly since habitual activity levels are difficult to measure.

Often, it is easier to detect the effects of inactivity than to measure it, both in terms of general health and physical fitness. Indoor rowing training is particularly well suited to improving both the physical fitness and physical activity levels of all individuals. For clarity, we will use the preferred definition of physical fitness, as used by health professionals, which is comprised of the following five essential components:

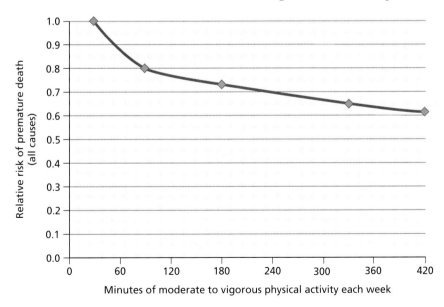

Fig 6.1 The risk of premature death decreases as a person's level of weekly physical activity increases (Source: 2008 Physical Activity Guidelines for Americans; www.health.gov)

1 Muscular strength
2 Muscular endurance
3 Cardiovascular health
4 Flexibility
5 Body composition

A person's overall physical fitness is then defined by how well they score in each separate fitness component. Researchers have measured the overall physical fitness of large samples of diverse adults and compared these to each person's daily

Strong evidence:

☒ Lower risk of early death

☒ Lower risk of coronary heart disease

☒ Lower risk of stroke

☒ Lower risk of high blood pressure

☒ Lower risk of adverse blood lipid profile

☒ Lower risk of type 2 diabetes

☒ Lower risk of metabolic syndrome

☒ Lower risk of colon cancer

☒ Lower risk of breast cancer

☒ Prevention of weight gain

☒ Weight loss, especially when combined with reduced calorie intake

☒ Improved cardiorespiratory and muscular fitness

☒ Prevention of falls

☒ Reduced depression

☒ Better cognitive function (for older adults)

Moderate to strong evidence:

☒ Better functional health (for older adults)

☒ Reduced obesity

Moderate evidence:

☒ Low risk of hip fracture

☒ Lower risk of lung cancer

☒ Lower risk of endometrial cancer

☒ Weight maintenance after weight loss

☒ Increased bone density

☒ Improved sleep quality

Fig 6.2 Health benefits from regular physical activity classified according to the current strength of scientific evidence. Physical activity in this context is considered activity that requires skeletal muscle activity and that elevates energy expenditure above-resting levels
(Source: 2008 Physical Activity Guidelines for Americans; www.health.gov)

activity levels. Unsurprisingly, the results show a direct relationship between regular physical activity levels and physical fitness. The individuals with high daily activity had the highest fitness levels, while the individuals with low daily activity had the lowest fitness levels. What has also become clear from research on this topic is that huge numbers of children and adults fail to achieve the minimum recommended amounts of physical activity needed for good health. Consequently, physical inactivity is now an acknowledged primary risk factor for many serious health problems including cardiovascular disease and obesity. Fortunately, there are substantial health benefits to increasing the amount of regular physical activity. Simply adding 90 minutes of moderate physical activity each week to a sedentary lifestyle will reduce the risk of premature death (see figure 6.1) by an impressive 20 per cent.

Figure 6.2 lists the various health benefits available from increased regular physical activity and is organised according to the strength of currently available scientific research. This already long list of confirmed health benefits is likely to become considerably longer over the next few decades as researchers identify more specific explanations as to why increases in physical activity levels promote longer and healthier lives.

Health professionals are working hard to find ways to reintroduce physical activity back into our daily lifestyles, but it is unlikely that the use of cars, lifts, washing machines and other labour-saving devices will diminish any time soon. The reality for most people is that dedicated periods of weekly time must be set aside to achieve the levels of physical activity needed for good health and fitness. Regular indoor rowing is one of the best ways to develop high levels of physical fitness and

physical activity. The specific and appropriate use of indoor rowing machines for this purpose is discussed later in this chapter in the section entitled 'Training for health'.

There are also growing numbers of adults who are specifically interested in training to improve indoor rowing performance. The usual focus of this training is the 2000m event, but there is also growing interest in other events, including the occasional 42.2km (26.2 miles) marathon event.

There are important differences between training for health versus training for performance. Competitive indoor rowing training is usually much more demanding than health focussed training, due largely to the use of higher amounts of specific indoor rowing training along with the need for progressive increases in weekly training loads. Competitive indoor rowers will typically exceed the minimum weekly physical activity recommendations for health benefits. Therefore, the training requirements for indoor rowers seeking improvements in indoor rowing performance are discussed separately in the section entitled 'Training for competitive performance'.

UNDERSTANDING THE KEY CONCEPTS OF EXERCISE TRAINING FOR HEALTH AND PERFORMANCE

Before describing the specific features of effective indoor rowing training for either health or competitive performance, it is important to understand several key training concepts. These concepts are the same for indoor rowing as they are for other types of exercise such as running, cycling, resistance training, on-water rowing, soccer or basketball.

PROGRESSIVE OVERLOAD

In order to improve the physical capability of the body, it is necessary to provide a stimulus that provides a significant physical challenge. For example, a 60kg 18-year-old woman can overload her current leg strength capabilities by performing repeated squat exercises while holding a 30kg weight bar. If this training stimulus is repeated at regular intervals for an indefinite number of weeks, her gains in leg strength will be impressive at first. However, as the weeks continue the gains will become smaller and smaller until leg strength eventually plateaus. At this point, additional strength gains can be produced by adding more weight to the bar (e.g. 5kg) to stimulate new physiological adaptations. This process is known as progressive overload and its appropriate application is essential to anyone who wants to improve the various fitness components rather than simply maintain a stable level.

SPECIFICITY

This concept refers to the phenomenon whereby the physiological effects of training are highly specific to the type of training undertaken. For example, training that provides an appropriate level of challenge to the cardiovascular system will mostly result in anatomical and physiological changes in the cardiovascular system, including the heart, lungs and blood. Similarly, strength training will only develop the individual muscle fibres that are recruited during training. The concept of specificity is of particular importance to competitive indoor rowers who wish to include cross-training activities in their regular training.

INDIVIDUALITY

This concept states that the effects of training will differ between individuals, even when they all follow the same standardised training programme. Research has shown that individual factors such as a person's genes and initial level of conditioning can alter the rate of fitness gains and influence the overall capacity of the body to adapt to training. A major research study recorded the fitness changes of 614 untrained adults who completed a 20 week indoor cycling programme. The average improvement in aerobic capacity was 18 per cent, but a small group of these adults achieved gains in excess of 40 per cent (high responders), while another small group achieved improvements of less than 5 per cent (low responders). An important implication of the individuality concept is that training benefits will be optimised when a person adheres to an exercise programme which has been adjusted to suit their individual needs and motivation.

RECOVERY

Recovery from training is critical to developing training adaptations. While exercise training provides the initial stimulus for changes in anatomy and physiology, it is only when adequate rest is provided in the hours and days following training that these changes occur. The effectiveness of the recovery period in promoting fitness gains is influenced by its duration as well as other important factors such as a person's diet and sleep quality.

Indoor rowing performance is strongly influenced by the amount of recovery applied between training sessions or before a major competition. The specific pattern of recovery incorporated into the final weeks of training before a major rowing competition is known as tapering. It is associated with additional improvements in 2000m performance of between 1 and 3 per cent.

REVERSIBILITY

This concept states that improvements in physical fitness and performance will decrease unless the overload stress is repeated at regular intervals. Typically, the stimulating effects of a single bout of cardiovascular or resistance exercise lasts for approximately 24 to 48 hours. After 48 hours, the anatomical and physiological adaptations of exercise training decrease unless further training is performed. Research suggests that most of the physiological adaptations from regular endurance training are lost within six weeks once training ends (detraining). Importantly, the loss of these adaptations is greatest in the first 3 to 14 days of detraining. It is especially difficult to construct a training programme that balances the need for appropriate recovery against the risk of allowing significant amounts of reversibility to occur.

TECHNIQUE

The specific technique that a person uses to achieve movement during exercise is an important training consideration. Poor stroke technique can limit the health and performance gains from indoor rowing training by reducing the overload stimulus or by developing ineffective muscle activation sequences. Since stroke technique is also important to the enjoyment, comfort and safety of an indoor rower, it is worth considering ways of improving technique when planning a comprehensive indoor rowing training programme for either health or performance.

UNDERSTANDING THE KEY COMPONENTS OF A TRAINING PROGRAMME

In order to help describe the type of training that will benefit indoor rowers, the overall training load can be separated according to the intensity, volume and frequency of individual sessions.

EXERCISE INTENSITY

This is how hard a person is actually working in terms of effort or energy expenditure. It can be described using subjective terms such as 'moderate' or 'vigorous' or through the use of a self-selected rating of perceived exertion (this is where a participant rates their level of exertion, usually using a score between 0 and 10, with 0 being a low level of exertion). More objectively, intensity can be quantified using absolute or relative measures. The absolute intensity of indoor rowing is commonly presented using power output (watts), speed (metres per second), pace (time over 500m) or rate of energy expenditure (kcal per hour). Relative exercise intensity is often supplied as a percentage of a person's maximum heart rate or aerobic power. Another relative intensity method, heart rate reserve, has gained popularity as a suitable way to prescribe exercise intensity when training for health (see figure 6.3, p. 58).

EXERCISE VOLUME

The volume of exercise refers to the amount of exercise performed. It is usually recorded as either the amount of time spent exercising (minutes), the distance covered (metres) or the total energy expenditure (kcal).

FREQUENCY

Frequency simply refers to how often exercise is performed and is usually measured by the number of exercise sessions completed each week.

Heart rate reserve is a useful method for monitoring and prescribing exercise intensity, especially when training for health gains. It requires a person to know both their maximum heart rate as well as their resting heart rate.

Resting heart rate should ideally be measured shortly after waking, before getting out of bed.

Maximum heart rate can be recorded (using a conventional wireless heart rate monitor) as the highest value obtained during a 2000m all-out effort or any indoor rowing activity which requires maximal effort for several minutes. Alternatively, maximum heart rate for indoor rowing can be estimated reasonably well using the formula:

☒ Maximum heart rate = 215 – Age (years)

Heart rate reserved is calculated as:

☒ Heart rate reserve = Maximum heart rate – Resting heart rate

Target heart rate for exercise is then calculated as:

☒ Target heart rate = Resting heart rate + Target % of heart rate reserve

Example:

Jane, a 55-year-old indoor rower with an interest in training for health, was advised by her doctor to exercise at 55 per cent of heart rate reserve. Her maximum heart rate during rowing is 160 beats per minute and her resting heart rate is 70 beats per minute, therefore, her heart rate reserve value is 90 beats per minute (i.e. 160–70). Her absolute heart rate at 55 per cent of heart rate reserve is then calculated as:

☒ Heart rate at 55 per cent of heart rate reserve = 70 + (55 per cent of 90) = 120 per minute

Fig 6.3 Calculating exercise intensity using the heart rate reserve method

THE IMPORTANCE OF PHYSICAL ACTIVITY FOR HEALTH

The effects of regular physical activity on improving health and longevity have been widely acknowledged for centuries. Nevertheless, the specific evidence that provides the necessary level of detail to support a therapeutic and health preserving role for physical activity has only become available in very recent years. While this may seem surprising, it must be appreciated that human health is an incredibly complex area of study. The amount of evidence required to make a conclusive and scientifically supported statement, such as 'regular exercise reduces a person's risk of developing heart disease' is immense.

The scale of the problem becomes obvious when specific questions about health and physical activity are considered. Does regular exercise help men and women who suffer with depression, digestive disorders, back pain, genetic linked diseases such as cystic fibrosis, as well as the many types of cancers? Are the benefits of exercise the same for young and old individuals, between men and women, for athletes and non-athletes, able-bodied and disabled individuals, pregnant women or obese men? It is far too convenient to assume that regular exercise will help all types of health problems or indeed that it may help at all. Exercise can even be an occasional source of health problems. For example, when a person engages in prolonged intense exercise, such as a marathon run, the ability of the immune system to resist infection is compromised for many hours after the event. This fact helps explain why marathon runners more frequently develop upper respiratory tract infections in the days immediately after a race than would otherwise be expected. The important point here is that while exercise is accepted as one of the very best ways to improve health and well-being, it is by no means a simple task to explain the benefits of exercise, or indeed the ways that a person can train to maximise the benefits of exercise.

Fortunately, there are now authoritative and clear answers to questions about the effects of exercise on human health, as well as training guidance to help achieve these benefits. These answers have been debated and agreed upon by expert panels of top scientists including medical experts, epidemiologists and exercise physiologists. The outcomes of these discussions have helped inform the physical activity policy statements of major health organisations and governments across the world (e.g. the World Health Organization; European Union). These statements include clear guidance regarding the volume, intensity and frequency of physical activity that is required for good health.

Currently, one of the best sources of physical activity guidance is the '2008 Physical Activity Guidelines for Americans' and these are the specific recommendations that we will use in this book. It should be noted that these guidelines are entirely consistent with government recommendations across Europe (including the governments of Ireland and the United Kingdom) and other parts of the world (e.g. Canada, Australia and New Zealand). In fact, the World Health Organization endorses the same physical activity guidelines for citizens throughout the world. By focussing on one particular set of guidelines, it is easier to provide readers with a clear and simple overview concerning the appropriate use of indoor rowing machines for optimising health gains.

WHAT IS THE RECOMMENDED AMOUNT OF ACTIVITY NEEDED TO GAIN SUBSTANTIAL HEALTH BENEFITS?

The recommended levels of weekly aerobic physical activity for most adults (aged 18 to 64 years) are displayed in figure 6.4. You should aim to complete a minimum of 150 minutes of moderate intensity aerobic physical activity every week. Keep in mind that you do not need to achieve this minimum amount of activity in your first weeks of training, especially if your current fitness levels are low. It is perfectly acceptable to start off with a lower level of activity and then progress gradually toward the 150 minute target. Also, the standard targets may not be appropriate for some older adults (age 65 and over) or individuals with particular health conditions (e.g. pregnant women, overweight and obese adults). For these special populations of adults, weekly physical activity targets may need to be adjusted (this issue is briefly discussed later in this chapter).

Initially, the targets may seem very high, possibly unachievable and unsustainable. However, it is essential to recognise that the recommended amounts can be achieved through the use of any combination of suitable aerobic physical activity. Indoor rowing is certainly one of the best methods to achieve the recommended amounts, but other activities such as cycling, swimming, walking, dance classes and even some household activities, such as pushing a lawnmower, can also be included as an effective supplement to indoor rowing.

WHAT DO MODERATE INTENSITY ACTIVITY AND VIGOROUS INTENSITY ACTIVITY ACTUALLY MEAN?

In order to make the guidelines as easy as possible to use, there are just two broad categories of exercise intensity that should be used. You can judge whether you are using either a moderate or vigorous intensity at any time during exercise by checking how easily you are able to talk, or by estimating how you feel on a scale of 0 to 10 (where 0 is sitting at rest and 10 is the highest effort possible) as follows:

☒ In order to achieve substantial health benefits from physical activity, these are the physical activity targets that you should try to achieve weekly:

    1. At least 150 minutes each week of moderate intensity aerobic physical activity OR

    2. At least 75 minutes each week of vigorous intensity aerobic physical activity OR

    3. A combination of 1 and 2

☒ For additional and extensive health benefits, weekly exercise targets can be increased to the following weekly activity targets:

    1. 300 minutes each week of moderate intensity aerobic physical activity OR

    2. 150 minutes each week of vigorous intensity aerobic physical activity OR

    3. A combination of 1 and 2

Fig 6.4 Weekly aerobic physical activity targets needed to achieve good health (Source: 2008 Physical Activity Guidelines for Americans; www.health.gov)

- moderate intensity is equivalent to a pace where you can talk comfortably but not sing. It is classified as a score of 5 or 6 (out of 10);
- vigorous intensity is equivalent to a pace where you can only say a few words before pausing for a breath. It is classified as a score of 7 or 8.

If you want to use a more objective way to check you are using an appropriate exercise intensity, then use the heart rate reserve method described in figure 6.3, along with a suitable heart rate monitor, to calculate the actual heart rate range needed for each intensity category. You will need to use the following information:

- moderate intensity exercise is classified as a heart rate reserve score between 45 and 65 per cent;
- vigorous intensity exercise is classified as a heart rate reserve between 65 and 84 per cent.

SELECTING YOUR WEEKLY LEVEL OF PHYSICAL ACTIVITY TARGET

You first need to decide what level of activity you ultimately want to achieve. Have a look at the information in figure 6.5 and consider which activity category best matches your ambitions and available time. Be careful to notice that the indicated number of minutes for each category is based on moderate intensity aerobic activity. If instead you plan to use vigorous

Levels of physical activity	Range of moderate-intensity minutes a week	Summary of overall health benefits	Comment
Inactive	No activity above baseline	None	Being inactive
Low	Activity beyond baseline but fewer than 150 minutes a week	Some	Low levels of activity are clearly preferable to an inactive lifestyle
Medium	150 minutes to 300 minutes a week	Substantial	Activity at the high end of the range has additional and more extensive health benefits than activity at the low end
High	More than 300 minutes a week	Additional	Current science does not allow researchers to identify an upper limit of activity above which there are no additional health benefits

Fig 6.5 Classification of total weekly physical activity into four separate categories (Source: 2008 Physical Activity Guidelines for Americans; www.health.gov)

aerobic activity, then you only need to achieve half as many minutes as necessary at moderate intensity: 2 minutes of moderate intensity aerobic activity provides similar health outcomes to 1 minute of vigorous intensity aerobic activity.

Hopefully, you will be able to work towards a medium level of physical activity or better. If a medium level of physical activity still seems too high, then just start off by doing as much as you feel you can. It is still much better to do some physical activity than to remain inactive. Just start slowly by using light to moderate aerobic activity for short periods (e.g. 5 minutes on the indoor rowing machine) and try to accumulate a little bit more exercise each week until you achieve the top of your comfort zone. As your training progresses, your fitness and confidence will improve, making it easier to achieve a medium level of activity. You may even find that it becomes possible to do significant amounts of weekly activity at a vigorous intensity. At this point, you could refocus your goals toward the high activity category, or remain in the medium activity category and consider using vigorous intensities to reduce total training time.

CHOOSING YOUR PREFERRED TYPES OF PHYSICAL ACTIVITY

We expect that many readers will want to use indoor rowing as their primary source of weekly aerobic physical activity and this is perfectly appropriate. But there are good reasons to regularly include other forms of physical activity into your training. Indeed, you are more likely to achieve the weekly activity totals over the course of a year when you also maintain a level of specific fitness for other activities such as swimming, cycling or hiking.

You can achieve superb health benefits from any form of aerobic activity, but indoor rowing is quite possibly the single best choice available. Enjoyment and motivation are easier to maintain when several choices of activity are available. For example, on an exceptionally nice day you will probably want to take full advantage of the good weather and while you may be able to take your rowing machine outside, you can't take it very far! Instead, why not make the most of the fitness that you have gained from regular indoor rowing by exploring a local forest or national park on foot or bike?

If indoor rowing is the only regular activity that you do, you may find it hard to maintain your weekly targets on the sporadic occasion when you decide to try a different activity. Good indoor rowing fitness may not be enough to compensate for a lack of specific fitness in alternative types of aerobic activity, causing a decrease in both the intensity and duration of the substitute activity. Keeping a decent level of specific fitness for other aerobic activities is also useful on occasions when you cannot use an indoor rowing machine, either because of practical limitations (e.g. travelling or holidaying in a remote location) or due to injury.

It is important to understand that while indoor rowing is a great all round activity, there are some health goals that indoor rowing machines are not well suited to improving. For example, an exclusive focus on indoor rowing is not the best idea for a person who wants to increase their bone health. Indoor rowing is a non-weight bearing sport and therefore has only minor effects on improving bone density and bone health. If a person is worried about their risk of developing osteoporosis or suffering a hip fracture, then it is worth including some weight bearing activity, such as walking, tennis or basketball into the overall training schedule.

Finally, we should point out that while the minimum recommended targets outlined above have exclusively focussed on aerobic activities, there are great benefits to other non-aerobic activities such as stretching and muscle strengthening exercises (e.g. weight-lifting or body circuits). This will provide additional health benefits and give balance to your training, especially if these supplemental forms of training are targeted toward the fitness components which are less stimulated during indoor rowing (e.g. strength training for chest muscles or flexibility for hamstring muscles). Even just a few minutes of regular stretching or strength training on alternate days can be enough to gain significant improvements. Adding balance to your training in this way may contribute to additional improvements in rowing technique, bone density and may even reduce your overall risk of injury.

SELECTING A WEEKLY STRUCTURE OF PHYSICAL ACTIVITY

You should separate your weekly activity target time into smaller time periods to divide across the week. Even if you could manage all 150 minutes of weekly moderate intensity activity in a single session, this would not provide the expected health and fitness benefits since you would lose many of the physiological adaptations between weekly sessions. Instead, improvements will be optimised when your weekly activity is spread more evenly across each week. An appropriate weekly structure is anything between three sessions per week, on alternate days, to training every day. Obviously, on a three session per week structure, the average length of each separate session will be 50 minutes and this may be too long for many people. If preferred, you can increase the number of weekly activity sessions to reduce the duration of each session. You can also use several sessions in a single day to help reduce session duration. For example, you might choose to do some activity in the morning and evening on the same day. Keep in mind that a single activity session should last at least 10 minutes.

There are many different ways to structure your weekly training to achieve excellent health benefits. The best structure will be the one that suits you and allows for a certain amount of flexibility. Start by trying out several different approaches to your weekly structure and see what you prefer. Prioritise the first few days of each week so that you get a good start on your weekly targets, this way you are less likely to feel squeezed for training time later in the week. If you do find yourself in that position, just complete your activity targets in a sensible fashion. Don't try anything dramatic, just do what you comfortably can and then start again the following week with renewed vigour. This will be far better for your overall enjoyment, comfort and adherence than substantially increasing your activity level in the final few days of the week only to sustain an injury or make the experience of training downright miserable. Have a look at the ways that other people have used indoor rowing to help achieve their weekly activity targets.

CASE STUDY

CLAIRE: AN ACTIVE MIDDLE-AGED WOMEN

Her goal and current activity pattern: Claire was a competitive on-water rower while at university but hasn't done any sort of structured activity for the past 20 years. She now wants to get back into shape using the indoor rowing machine that she recently purchased. Her job is mainly office-based work but she walks continuously for at least 20 minutes each day.

Starting out: Claire begins her first week by adding 20 minutes of moderate intensity rowing on three different days. She plans to do more indoor rowing, and to gradually replace the moderate intensity activity with vigorous activity.

Making good progress: Every two weeks, Claire adds an extra 5 minutes of moderate intensity rowing to each session until she is able to complete 40 minutes per session. She then switches to four indoor rowing sessions per week, with each session lasting 30 minutes. Two of these sessions start with 5 minutes of moderate intensity rowing followed by 25 minutes of vigorous intensity rowing. The other two sessions are performed at moderate intensity for 40 minutes each.

Reaching her goal: Eventually, Claire completes 5 days per week, including a session of indoor rowing that lasts for one hour (30 minutes at moderate intensity, 5 minute rest, 30 minutes of vigorous intensity). She also goes swimming for 40 minutes on alternate weekends.

CASE STUDY

MARTIN: AN INACTIVE MIDDLE-AGED MAN

His goal and current activity pattern: Martin works as a home shopping delivery driver and wants to become a regular indoor rower. He and his wife have recently joined a local gym and they usually take a 50 minute walk on most weekends.

Starting out: Martin starts a combined indoor rowing and indoor cycling programme with his wife. On his first week, he does four separate sessions in the gym, including 10 minutes of rowing and 10 minutes of cycling, all at a moderate intensity.

Making good progress: He gradually develops his rowing technique and comfort levels and progresses to 30 minutes of moderate intensity rowing on each of the four sessions that he completes at the gym. He also goes cycling for 40 minutes in the morning on one of his days off.

Reaching his goal: After four months, he decides to join the Concept2 million metre club (an online achievement recognition scheme organised by Concept2). He now rows on most days with a session usually lasting between 30 and 90 minutes and plans to join his local on-water rowing club once he has reached the one million metre target.

CONSIDERATIONS FOR SPECIAL POPULATIONS

As mentioned earlier, the recommended minimum amount of 150 minutes of moderate intensity aerobic activity may be unsuitable for certain groups of adults with health conditions that require specialist medical advice. In many of these cases, it will be appropriate to use a lower weekly physical activity target. The following comments are provided as general guidance only.

OLDER ADULTS (65+ YEARS OF AGE)

The benefits of regular physical activity for individuals aged 65 and older are substantial. However, this is also the least active age group and individual physical abilities can vary considerably. All adults in this age group will have experienced some loss of physical fitness and many will also have chronic conditions or physical disabilities that restrict their capacity for physical activity.

Regular indoor rowing is an excellent choice of activity for this age group, especially when combined with other activities such as balance training, strength training and flexibility development. The guidelines provided in figure 6.6 are physical activity recommendations for older adults.

For older adults who are physically healthy and have no major health restrictions, the recommendations for physical activity provided in figure 6.4 (see p. 60) are generally appropriate. Older adults may find it more enjoyable to use moderate rather than vigorous intensity activity. However, it is worth noting that indoor rowing competitions are popular with older adults, including individuals who are over the age of 100 years! Clearly, vigorous intensity indoor rowing may be appropriate for some older adults, but this is a decision that requires consultation with a general practitioner or personal physician.

The guidelines below are just for older adults (aged 65 and older).

☒ When older adults cannot do 150 minutes of moderate intensity aerobic activity a week because of chronic conditions, they should be as physically active as their abilities and condition allows.

☒ Older adults should do exercise that maintains or improves balance if they are at risk of falling.

☒ Older adults should determine their level of effort for physical activity relative to their level of fitness.

☒ Older adults with chronic conditions should understand whether and how their conditions affect their ability to undertake regular physical activity safely.

Fig 6.6 Recommended physical activity targets for older adults
(Source: 2008 Physical Activity Guidelines for Americans; www.health.gov)

PREGNANCY AND POST PREGNANCY

Moderate physical activity is recommended for pregnant women and in the period after birth. Scientific evidence has shown that there is no added risk of low birth weight or pregnancy loss when women perform regular moderate intensity during pregnancy. There is even evidence to suggest that physically active women have a lower risk of complications during pregnancy and may experience a reduction in the duration of labour. Importantly, regular activity can help control excessive maternal weight gain, both during pregnancy and in the months after giving birth.

Women who are already regularly active at the start of pregnancy can continue to follow the standard guidance of a minimum of 150 minutes of moderate intensity aerobic activity. The effects of using vigorous intensity activity during pregnancy have not been well studied. There are some suggestions that the higher maternal body temperatures experienced during vigorous intensity may have detrimental effects on foetal development. Given that there are extensive benefits from the use of moderate intensity activity during pregnancy, current recommendations advise that pregnant women prefer the use of moderate rather than vigorous intensity activity. Once pregnancy is complete, women can slowly resume regular activity using the standard recommendations for all adults. Regular activity in the postpartum period does not appear to adversely affect breast milk or infant growth and development.

Indoor rowing is usually suitable for use during pregnancy, providing that it remains comfortable for the mother and is not performed in hot ambient environments ($\geq 25°C$). Once stroke length is significantly reduced, or the rowing action becomes uncomfortable, it is better to use alternative forms of physical activity, such as recumbent cycling. After giving birth, it is usually possible and safe to resume indoor rowing training after approximately six to eight weeks. When training does resume, it is especially important to begin slowly since a significant amount of detraining is likely to have occurred. In all cases, decisions about physical activity levels, both during pregnancy and in the postpartum period, should only be taken after consultation with an appropriately qualified medical specialist. This is of particular importance for women who want to start regular exercise during pregnancy.

OVERWEIGHT AND OBESE ADULTS

There is extensive and detailed evidence to show that regular amounts of either moderate or vigorous physical activity are helpful for controlling body weight in overweight (body mass index of $25.0–29.9$ kg/m^2) and obese individuals (body mass index of ≥ 30.0 kg/m^2), both for preventing additional weight gain and for assisting weight loss. There is also impressive evidence to show that overweight and obese individuals who have good aerobic fitness typically enjoy better health, well-being and longevity in comparison with overweight and obese individuals who have low aerobic fitness. While there is a compelling case to encourage weight loss in overweight and obese adults, recent medical reports have also raised concerns that repeated episodes of weight cycling are actually detrimental to health. Weight cycling is the process of losing and subsequently regaining large amounts of body weight. Recent reports are beginning to challenge many of the conventional beliefs regarding the relationship between a person's body weight and their general health.

In order for a person to lose body fat and body weight, they must first develop an 'energy deficit' whereby fewer calories are consumed than expended by the body. Interestingly, the loss of body fat and body weight is similar when weight loss is achieved through dietary restriction alone or through a combination of dietary restriction and aerobic exercise, providing that the total energy deficit achieved in each treatment is similar. In other words, the effectiveness of a weight reduction intervention depends on the size of energy deficit achieved rather than the method used to develop the energy deficit. In theory, this suggests that dietary or physical activity interventions should be equally effective for weight reduction. However, in practical terms, it is extremely difficult for overweight and obese individuals to generate a large daily energy deficit using just physical activity alone. This is because most overweight and obese adults also have low physical fitness, at least at the start of an activity intervention, which limits the amount and intensity of activity possible. Actual rates of weekly weight loss are typically much lower for standard aerobic activity interventions (approximately 0.2kg body weight loss per week) when compared to typical energy restricted diets (approximately 0.8kg body weight loss per week).

At first glance, the faster rates of weight reduction with dietary restriction might suggest that physical activity strategies are of lesser importance. However, most weight loss studies have been conducted over relatively short periods of six months or less. When comparisons are made over longer periods of between one and two years, individuals who use aerobic-based physical activity interventions frequently have better long-term weight loss success and experience fewer episodes of weight cycling. These interesting findings are partly explained by evidence that appetite is stimulated less when energy deficits are achieved through physical activity interventions rather than through diet restriction. The best results from weight loss interventions tend to be achieved through the combined use of regular physical activity and diet modification.

Indoor rowing machines provide an excellent way for overweight and obese individuals to achieve weekly physical activity targets. However, some individuals may need to complete more physical activity than normally recommended to achieve their desired weight loss or weight control targets, possibly requiring between 150 and 300 minutes of moderate intensity activity per week. In order to successfully achieve these higher levels of weekly activity, it is usually necessary to supplement indoor rowing with other activities such as cycling and walking. It is especially important to start slowly and then gradually increase the total amount of weekly activity as fitness levels progress. In the first weeks after starting regular physical activity, it is perfectly acceptable to select either low or moderate intensity activity and to exercise for less than 150 minutes per week (if necessary). While this may be initially frustrating, the gains in fitness and subsequent improvement in exercise tolerance can happen relatively quickly, which provides additional motivation to increase physical activity levels.

FURTHER INFORMATION ON PHYSICAL ACTIVITY

There is plenty of additional information available at the following excellent websites (including further details about physical activity targets for special populations and helpful suggestions on how to achieve your personal activity targets):

- United Kingdom: http://www.nhs.uk/livewell/fitness/pages/howmuchactivity.aspx
- Ireland: http://www.getirelandactive.ie/
- United States: http://www.health.gov/paguidelines/default.aspx
- New Zealand: http://www.moh.govt.nz/moh.nsf/indexmh/physicalactivity
- Australia: http://www.health.gov.au/internet/main/publishing.nsf/Content/health-pubhlth-strateg-phys-act-guidelines
- Canada: http://www.csep.ca/english/View.asp?x=587
- Global recommendations from the World Health Organization (WHO): http://www.who.int/dietphysicalactivity/en/index.html

TRAINING FOR COMPETITIVE PERFORMANCE

This section presents helpful information that can be used to develop an effective training approach for improving 2000m indoor rowing performance. This information is based on our own experiences of training indoor and on-water rowers, from examination of the training programmes used by highly successful indoor rowers and from relevant scientific research. The details are most appropriate for the needs of dedicated indoor rowers, but are also relevant to on-water rowers who have chosen to add a specific training goal for indoor rowing performance. In both situations, it is important to appreciate the need for individualisation of training loads.

The most effective training scenario is one where each session is adapted to the rower's individual performance features. These include a rower's base fitness and skill levels, unique rates of physiological, psychological and technical adaptation as well as their commitment and available training time. Unfortunately, it is beyond the scope of any book to provide highly detailed training recommendations that meet this individualisation requirement. Instead, we hope that each reader will be able to use the essential information in this section to create a unique and successful approach to indoor rowing training.

SELECTING YOUR 2000M TARGETS AND USING TIME TRIALS

It is important to make a clear estimate of the target level of 2000m performance that you want to achieve. Ideally, this estimate should be established before training starts but, if this is not possible, it is acceptable to identify a 2000m target during the early phase of training. Many indoor rowers will already have a reasonable idea of their starting fitness at the point that they decide to start training and this can help estimate a suitable 2000m performance target. Typically, these estimates are reasonably good when made by individuals who have six months or more of prior indoor rowing experience, including several successful 2000m efforts.

For individuals with limited experience of competitive indoor rowing, it is often valuable to complete a 2000m time trial soon after training has commenced, possibly once six weeks of regular training has been accomplished. This will give a good estimate of baseline fitness levels and introduces new indoor rowers to the demands of 2000m racing. It is not strictly necessary to perform this time trial at maximal effort and doing so can sometimes be disheartening to a rower if the outcome does not meet initial performance hopes. The idea of using this approach for the initial time trial is that it allows a person to perform at near-maximal effort, possibly around 95 per cent of capacity, in order to gain valuable information without reaching the point of complete exhaustion. However, the nature of competitive indoor rowing training is extremely challenging and this is something that all successful rowers must ultimately come to accept, irrespective of whether they chose to perform a time trial at maximal or near maximal intensity.

Keep in mind that the better your initial 2000m performance score, the less likely you are to experience a large increase in performance by the end of the training period. For example, a healthy 20-year-old male (90kg) who can pull a 6:10 (6 minutes 10 seconds) on a Concept2 machine at the start of training would be fortunate to reduce this time by 10 seconds or more by the end of a training season. However, another male of similar age and weight who achieves 8:00 at the start of training is quite likely to experience a large increase in performance of 20 to 60 seconds or better. You can get a good idea of what is reasonably possible for your own age, sex and weight by consulting the appropriate online rankings (http://www.concept2.com/sranking03/rankings.asp). Have a look at the typical range of performance times and the percentile rankings to gain an understanding of the average performance level (i.e. 50th percentile). Doing so will provide a decent approximation of the results that can reasonably be expected after six months or more of appropriate indoor rowing training.

It is valuable to attempt 2000m tests at regular intervals. This will provide an update on your rate of progress and allows suitable adjustments to training intensity to be made. It is also a good way to prepare for indoor racing because it gives each rower a chance to develop the necessary familiarity and confidence to sustain a high intensity rowing effort for between 6 and 10 minutes. Regular 2000m time trials or indoor races also provide opportunities to try different psychological, nutritional and pace strategies. A suitable interval between 2000m attempts is six weeks. This time period is usually long enough for most rowers to gain a noticeable improvement in performance as a result of the training induced physiological adaptations. If you think you might benefit from a more frequent use of time trials, then consider an alternative trial length (e.g. 250m, 1000m, 5000m, 6000m, 30 minutes or 60 minutes). These time trial durations are especially useful when matched to the specific emphasis in a particular training phase. For example, a 60 minute time trial is useful during an endurance development phase, whereas a 250m test is best used during the high intensity competitive phase of training.

Lastly, consider treating the days and hours before a time trial in much the same way as you would before a real race. Pay attention to your nutrition and hydration status and also consider setting out a special race day warm-up to use before time trials. This will help make the time trials feel more authentic and can improve trial performance. The sense of familiarity that comes from preparing for time trials in this way can be helpful for controlling anxiety levels before actual competition.

MAKING GOOD USE OF YOUR TIME

In addition to measuring your 2000m performance, you need to think carefully about the amount of training time that you can dedicate to actual indoor rowing each week. Generally, the more time you can dedicate to regular indoor rowing, the better your performance improvement. It is important to understand that performance gains are likely to be greatest when most of your available training time is dedicated to the specific task of indoor rowing.

There is no direct evidence from scientific studies to support superior gains in 2000m performance when indoor rowers replace specific training activity time (i.e. indoor rowing) with non-specific training activity (e.g. weight training, cycling or core stability training). Researchers have not yet directed significant efforts to this question. Indeed, it may surprise readers to learn that there is practically no research evidence that provides direct support for the idea that 2000m rowing performance (indoor or on-water rowing) improves when weight lifting is included in a training programme, despite the widespread popularity of this practice. The alleged benefits are almost entirely based on practical experience or from theoretical expectations. But there is certainly good reason to believe this, and related evidence supports performance enhancement from the appropriate use of a select range of non-specific training activities. This case is strongest when non-specific rowing training is used as a supplement to specific rowing training, rather than substituted for existing training time. The potential gains in 2000m performance from the addition of supplemental non-specific rowing activity, are at best, likely to be small and do require a greater overall investment of time that may not suit many indoor rowers. As a general rule, the more time that can be committed to specific indoor rowing training, the better the likely gain in 2000m performance. That said, there are still specific individual circumstances where the use of non-specific training activity is extremely valuable, independent of whether such activities will directly enhance 2000m indoor rowing performance.

All highly successful indoor rowers will have spent many hours training to achieve their results. Truly world class 2000m ergometer performances are usually only achieved by individuals once they have completed at least 24 months of indoor rowing training, at which point, between 1000 and 2000 hours of training have usually been performed on the rowing machine (approximately 10 to 20 hours per week). In exceptional cases, world class indoor rowing performances have been achieved by individuals after shorter periods of specific training. However, these individuals usually started competitive indoor rowing with well-established pedigrees in other competitive sports, typically endurance based sports. While it would be fascinating to discover the amount of 2000m performance improvement possible if the average indoor rower was able to complete 10 to 20 hours of training each week, in practice this sort of time commitment is unrealistic. Most indoor rowers perform very well on a weekly training allowance of between two and six hours.

UNDERSTANDING TRAINING INTENSITY

While the concept of training intensity is easy to understand, different exercise intensities will stimulate different physiological adaptations and have an important influence on the rate of improvement in 2000m performance. If exercise intensity is too low, no adaptations will take place and rowing performance is unlikely to change. But when indoor rowing is performed for sufficient duration at either moderate or high intensities, a range of suitable physiological adaptations occur. The extent to which any specific physiological adaptation develops will depend on the specific intensity used. Figure 6.7 presents the range of effective training intensities commonly used for indoor rowing training. It is important to recognise that the relative distribution of exercise intensity during a single week of training is largely determined by the phase of training, but generally most indoor rowing training (expressed either as time or distance completed) is performed at intensity Category 5 (low to moderate intensity), with the least training time performed at Category 1 (maximum intensity).

ADDING STRUCTURE TO INDOOR ROWING TRAINING WITH A PERIODISED APPROACH

An important feature of effective indoor rowing training is the use of a periodised approach. Basically, periodisation is based on the idea that the physiological abilities and technical skills necessary for competition are best improved when a training programme is structured into distinct 'periods' of training time. These periods can be

Intensity category	Description of intensity	Approximate competitive pace	Stroke rates (typical)*	Heart rate (% of maximum)	Sample workout (basic structure)
5	Low to moderate	Marathon pace to half-marathon pace	16 to 22	65% to 85%	3 x 30 minutes (minutes 0–10 stroke rate 18, minutes 10–20 at rate 20, minutes 20–30 at rate 22) with 5 minute rest break between 30 minute section
4	Moderate to high	5000m race pace to one hour time trial pace	22 to 28	85% to 95%	[5 minute warm-up of easy rowing] 3 x15 minutes (minutes 0–5 at rate 24, minutes 5–10 at rate 26, minutes 10–15 at rate 28) with 8 minute rest break between 15 minute section [5 minute cool-down of easy rowing]
3	High	2000m race pace	28 to 34	95% to 100%	[10 minute warm-up] 4 x 1000m with 3 to 6 minutes of active rest between each 1000m effort (low intensity rowing) [5 minute cool-down]
2	Very high	1000m race pace	32 to 38	100%	[10 minute warm-up] 6 x 500m with 1.5 to 3 minutes of active rest between each 500m effort (low intensity rowing) [5 minute cool-down]
1	Maximum intensity	250m race pace	>36	100%	[10 minute warm-up] 8 x 100m with full recovery (>3 minutes) between each 100m effort [10 minute cool-down]

Fig 6.7 Range of suitable training intensities for indoor rowing (*Assumes use of a stationary rowing machine with standard resistance settings. If a dynamic/sliding machine is used, strokes rates will be approximately two strokes per minute higher)

organised into separate 'phases', which vary in duration from a few weeks to many months. Each phase has its own set of specific physiological and skill based objectives.

While there have been many refinements and adjustments to periodisation terminology over the years, in this book, we will use the conventional terms and sequence of phases as follows:

1 Preparation phase
2 Competition phase
3 Transition phase

1. Preparation phase

The preparation phase provides the foundation of any training programme and is designed to provide the basic physiological, technical and psychological adaptations needed to cope with the more challenging training that follows later in the season. It is the longest phase of training and usually occupies 50 per cent or more of total training time. In the specific case of endurance sports, such as indoor rowing, progressive overload in the preparation phase is provided through gradual increases in weekly training volume, while peak training volume is typically reached toward the end of the preparation phase. Increases in relative training intensity (i.e. intensity relative to current performance capability) are usually introduced later in the preparation phase to further increase training load, but it is noteworthy that absolute intensity (i.e. power or pace display) increases throughout the entire preparation phase in line with fitness gains. Current training theory suggests that this conservative approach to early season training results in superior overall gains in performance

later in the season. The important training objectives typically achieved in the preparation phase for indoor rowing are listed in the box below.

Objectives achieved

- Cardiovascular changes to enhance VO_2max
  - Increasing heart size and strength
  - Increasing blood volume and red cell volume
  - Increasing haemoglobin content
- Muscular changes
  - Increasing size of individual muscle fibres
  - Increasing aerobic capacity of muscle fibres
  - Increasing the size and number of capillaries surrounding muscle fibres
- Ventilation changes
  - Developing a coordinated breathing pattern where each inhalation starts at the finish of the stroke
- Developing injury resistance and core strength
  - Strengthening tendons and connective tissue
  - Addressing any strength imbalance
- Skill demands
  - Improving stroke to stroke consistency and stroke smoothness
  - Improving sequencing of body segments
  - Increasing efficiency of power transfer from legs, back and arms into handle force
  - Developing a relaxed, effective stroke profile that avoids unnecessary movements

2. Competition phase

The competition phase is designed to provide specific preparation for indoor racing and should normally last about eight weeks. Training volume usually decreases during the competition phase to make way for significant increases in relative training intensity. Interval training at, or above, 2000m race pace provides the main source of progressive overload in this phase. Ideally, preparation for a major indoor rowing event should include several indoor races of lesser importance during the competition phase. In practice, this is often difficult for indoor rowers since there may not be many indoor rowing events in the local area.

In the final days or weeks of the competition phase, it is normal to include a period of tapering. Tapering refers to the process whereby training volume is reduced in a controlled manner. The duration of the taper will depend on both the training load and total period of training. As a general rule, a long taper (two to three weeks) will only be appropriate for indoor rowers who have sustained high training loads for many months, usually achieving 80km or more per week. Indoor rowers who typically perform comparatively low training volumes (e.g. 15 to 30km per week) usually only benefit from minor reductions in training volume during the 2–3 days before competition. During a period of tapering, the intensity of training should be maintained at pre-taper levels. The issue of tapering is discussed again at the end of this chapter.

3. Transition phase

The transition phase follows the competition phase and usually lasts four weeks or more. This phase is effectively a period of non-specific training designed to allow the indoor rower's body to recover and rejuvenate from the accumulated physical and psychological stresses of training. In fact, it is common to stop indoor rowing entirely and to switch to aerobic cross-training activities such as cycling, kayaking or running. This helps maintain general fitness levels and provides an opportunity to resolve any persistent minor rowing-related injuries. The exclusive use of cross-training activities in the transition phase reduces the risk of developing overuse injuries, particularly in the wrists, ribs and lower back regions, once regular indoor rowing training begins again.

It is also useful to take a psychological break from indoor rowing, especially after many months of dedicated training. The key to a successful transition phase is a significant reduction in both the volume and intensity of any training that is performed. Many indoor rowers prefer to include some specific indoor rowing activity during this phase and this is perfectly acceptable providing that low training loads are selected. Similarly, many indoor rowers will benefit from time off from regular rowing machine use and frequently gain a welcome increase in motivation to begin another competitive season.

An understanding of each of the above points will help you to detect the underlying structure contained in the example indoor rowing training programme that follows in the next section. The ability to recognise the important structural features used in a periodised training approach will make it relatively easy for an indoor rower to plan their own individualised training activities.

DEVELOPING A COMPREHENSIVE TRAINING APPROACH

Periodised training programmes can be further divided into separate training units known as microcycles (small), mesocycles (medium) and macrocycles (large). There is no agreement about how long each cycle should last, but each one should reveal a regular and repetitive pattern of applied overload. Macrocycles are any large unit of training time, where 'large' typically refers to either the entire training season or the separate phases within a season (i.e. preparation, competition and transition). Each macrocycle consists of separate mesocycles which are described as medium sized units of training. Each mesocycle usually has its own set of broad training objectives (e.g. strength development, speed development). These usually last between two and six weeks and are composed of smaller units of time known as microcycles. Ultimately, it is the arrangement and construction of each microcycle that provides the backbone of a training programme.

Figure 6.8 shows two different 7 day microcycles. The overall training load is the same in both cases even though the distribution of the training load differs. Notice the way that both examples show a smooth training progression with one rest/low load day of training each week. The same microcycle can then be reapplied in subsequent weeks with or without an increase in the overall training load. Since progressive overload is important to stimulating performance gains, any additional weekly training load can be evenly spread across all training sessions using the established microcycle structure. These principles can also be used to sequence two or more microcycles into a mesocycle (see figure 6.9).

The use of a cycled approach within a periodised training programme helps to establish a regular training pattern that is easy to adjust to meet the recovery requirements of an individual athlete. In theory, this will improve the quality of

Summary

In review, the key points from the discussion on training phases are summarised below:

- Training load is determined by the volume and intensity of training performed.
- Physiological adaptations are stimulated when training loads provide sufficient overload in the target areas of the body.
- Progressive overload can be used to promote sustained gains in physiological adaptations over many months of training
- Competitive indoor rowers develop progressive overload in their training by gradual increases in training volume and intensity.
- The typical pattern of progressive overload used by indoor rowers begins with a steady increase in training volume. At a later stage, the progressive overload is further developed though an increase in relative training intensity.
- Time periods of extended recovery must be provided at regular points in the training programme to allow for consolidation of physiological and performance gains.

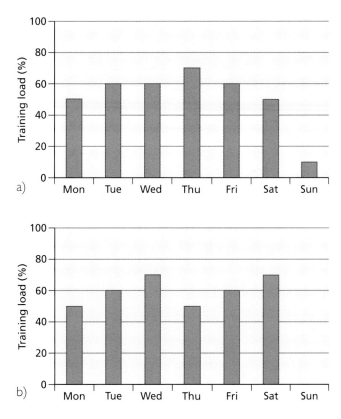

Fig 6.8 a) Example of a loading pattern for a single peak microcycle b) Example of a loading pattern for a double peak microcycle

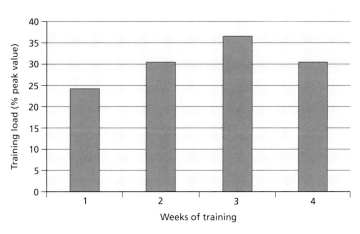

Fig 6.9 Example of loading pattern for a mesocycle

Note

Training load has been calculated as Volume × Intensity using the adjustment factors for each of the five intensity categories in figure 6.7, p. 71 (Intensity 5 = 0.2; Intensity 4 = 0.4; Intensity 3 = 0.6; Intensity 2 = 0.8; Intensity 1 = 1.0). Although these values are somewhat arbitrary, they do provide a reasonable indication of the stress on the body which is consistently applied across the full training plan.

training and enhance the rate of adaptation. It should also reduce injury risk by avoiding the abrupt changes in training load that are often associated with various injuries. Furthermore, a periodised programme with defined loading cycles improves the implementation of a technique development plan. Skill based rowing training can be routinely assigned to sessions with low overall training load, allowing for better concentration and focus. Both the rate of learning as well as the retention of new skills will benefit from this structured approach. Lastly, since we are all creatures of habit, it is much easier to balance lifestyle and training demands with periodised training. For example, an indoor rower is less likely to skip dinner or stay up late on a Monday night if they are well aware of the high intensity interval session that takes place on Tuesday mornings.

THEORY TO PRACTICE: BUILDING A PERIODISED PROGRAMME FOR A COMPETITIVE INDOOR ROWER

In order to explain how the various aspects of periodisation theory can be applied to a particular individual, we have constructed a 26 week training programme based on standard periodisation principles. We developed this programme based on the needs of a healthy 30-year-old man (80kg) who began indoor rowing around three months before the start of this programme. His goal was to compete at the National Indoor Rowing Championships (in the 2000m category), which was scheduled for the last day of this training programme (Sunday of week 26). A time trial at the start of training revealed a baseline 2000m performance ability of 7 minutes 23 seconds and his goal for the national championships was 6 minutes 40 seconds. He was willing to complete a maximum of five hours of training each week, if necessary. At the completion of this training programme, he achieved a personal best performance of 6 minutes 35 seconds at the National Championships.

Figure 6.10 shows the overall progression of training load and training volume during the preparation phase (18 weeks) and competition phase (8 weeks) leading up to the major indoor rowing event at the end of the training period. The progression of training intensity is presented separately in figure 6.11.

Sample training plans that correspond to the volume and intensity targets for weeks 3, 13 and 23 are presented in figures 6.12, 6.14 and 6.16, respectively. The daily training load is presented separately in figures 6.13 (week 3), 6.15 (week 13) and 6.17 (week 23) to show the pattern of distribution across each week.

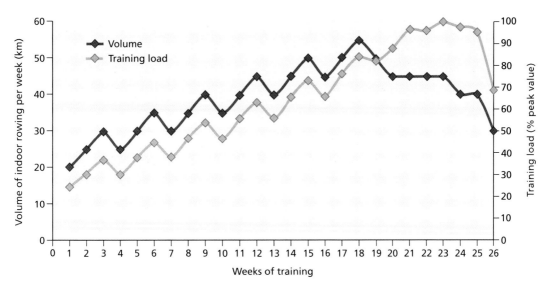

Fig 6.10 Overview of a 26 week periodised training programme suitable for a competitive indoor rower training for a 2000m race. Weekly training volume and training load are displayed.

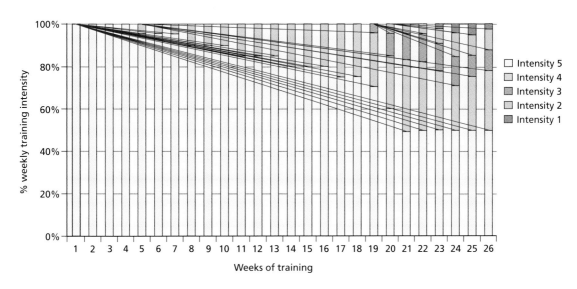

Fig 6.11 Overview of a 26 week periodised training programme suitable for a competitive indoor rower in training for their first 2000m event. Weekly training intensity is displayed using intensity categories 1 to 5, where category 1 is defined as low to moderate intensity and category 5 is defined as maximal intensity (see figure 6.7, p. 71, for more details of these intensity categories)

Day	Session
Monday	
Tuesday	6km of continuous rowing at 'Intensity 5' with focus on consistent power per stroke
Wednesday	5km of continuous rowing at 'Intensity 5' with focus on controlling seat movement in recovery phase
Thursday	5km of continuous rowing at 'Intensity 5'-stroke rate changes each 1km (e.g. 16–18–20–18–16)
Friday	
Saturday	6km of continuous rowing at 'Intensity 5' with focus on body posture
Sunday	8km of rowing at 'Intensity 5' but with a 5 minute stretching break after 4km

Fig 6.12 Example of the week 3 training schedule for a novice indoor rower (weekly totals: volume = 30km; intensity = 100% at intensity category 5)

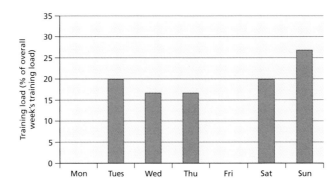

Fig 6.13 Distribution of weekly training load for week 3 training for a novice indoor rower

Day	Session
Monday	5km of continuous rowing at 'Intensity 5' with sections of 'eyes closed' rowing 50 strokes after each 1km
Tuesday	2km at 'Intensity 5' then 2 x 3km at 'Intensity 4' (rates of 24–26–28 for each 1km; repeated) with 6 minute rest interval
Wednesday	5km of continuous rowing at 'Intensity 5' with focus on pushing with even pressure on both legs
Thursday	8km of rowing at 'Intensity 5' but with 5 minute stretching break after 4km
Friday	
Saturday	6km of continuous rowing at 'Intensity 5' (rates of 18–20–22–18–20–22 to match each km of rowing)
Sunday	8km of continuous rowing at 'Intensity 5' with focus on keeping a relaxed grip on handles, especially towards the end

Fig 6.14 Example of the week 13 training schedule for a novice indoor rower (weekly totals: volume = 40km; intensity = 85% at intensity category 5 and 15% at intensity category 4)

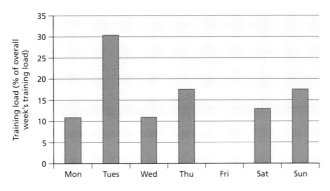

Fig 6.15 Distribution of weekly training load for week 13 training for a novice indoor rower

Day	Session
Monday	2km at 'Intensity 5' then 4 x 250m and 1 x 125m at 'Intensity 1' with 4 minute rest then 2km at 'Intensity 5'
Tuesday	1km at 'Intensity 5' then 4 x 1500km and 1 x 750m at 'Intensity 3' with 7 minute rest then 1km at 'Intensity 5'
Wednesday	1 x 8km at 'Intensity 5'
Thursday	1 x 8km at 'Intensity 4'
Friday	
Saturday	2km at 'Intensity 5' then 3 x 750m at 'Intensity 2' with 5 minute rest then 2km at 'Intensity 5'
Sunday	4.5km at 'Intensity 5' then 4.375km at 'Intensity 4'

Fig 6.16 Example of the week 23 training schedule for a novice indoor rower
(weekly totals: volume = 45km; intensity = 50% at intensity category 5, 27.5% at intensity category 4, 15% at intensity category 3, 5% at intensity category 2 and 2.5% at intensity category 1)

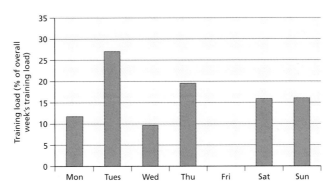

Fig 6.17 Distribution of weekly training load for week 23 training of a novice indoor rower

Summary

Many indoor rowers, especially beginners, fail to structure their training and often try to do as much as possible in whatever training time is available. Instead of using a periodised approach, these rowers end up turning each training session into a race. Although the initial gains in performance are often impressive, the rate of improvement quickly becomes unsustainable, at which point the rowers usually lose their enthusiasm to continue training. The use of a periodised approach to session planning helps ensure that progressive overload is applied throughout the training period. This will make it possible to enjoy continued gains in short- and long-term indoor rowing performance while reducing the risk of injury and burnout. Most importantly, the variety that a periodised programme offers makes training much more enjoyable and provides ample opportunity for each indoor rower to make changes to suit personal needs and preferences. The 26 week periodised training programme that we presented above represents a cautious introduction to competitive indoor rowing training. However, once you have some experience of the benefits of using a periodised approach, the next step is to make your own periodised programme that better matches your unique training requirements and performance objectives. At this point, you are likely to find added benefits to using a more aggressive approach to training, especially if you are willing to use higher training volumes and intensities. The final section of this chapter includes a selection of eight training tips which are useful to keep in mind when developing your own training programme.

EIGHT TRAINING TIPS FOR COMPETITIVE INDOOR ROWERS

1. START GRADUALLY

The first weeks of indoor rowing training can easily be among the toughest, especially for new rowers or rowers returning after an extended break from regular training. The first strokes of each session usually feel fine, probably even quite comfortable, and may even make you wonder why you didn't do this sooner. Nevertheless, if a sensible pace is not selected, discomfort quickly follows and the handle will probably end up back where it started – in the storage position!

The first weeks of training should simply be a gentle introduction to regular indoor rowing with the main aim of developing a regular activity pattern. By starting sessions gradually, keeping both the length and intensity of each session short and easy, indoor rowers are less likely to drop out of training and more likely to develop a keen enthusiasm for regular training. Fitness gains should become apparent within the first weeks of training but are most likely to be noticed during actual training. The likely gains include improvements in comfort levels at a set rowing pace (e.g. 2:30/500m) and increases in endurance capacity, as indicated by an increase in total rowing time or distance completed during each session.

It is far better to end a training session with plenty of energy to spare and avoid abrupt finishing spurts. This stable approach is much better for keeping an indoor rower's enthusiasm for future training sessions, whereas sessions that end with sprint finishes are often remembered for being more difficult than they actually were and this can be an unwelcome memory when considering whether to start the subsequent session. The gradual approach to starting indoor rowing training may seem needlessly conservative, but it is very effective in keeping training motivation high and improving exercise adherence.

2. DEVELOP AND SUSTAIN A BASE OF ENDURANCE WORK

The majority of an indoor rower's energy requirement for training and competition comes from the aerobic energy system and the most suitable way to develop aerobic adaptations is lots of moderate intensity indoor rowing. In addition to developing important cardiovascular and muscular adaptations, prolonged moderate intensity rowing is also a very good way to develop stroke technique. For competitive indoor rowers, it is worth noting that the training practices of competitive on-water rowers have evolved over many decades to emphasise high volumes of base endurance work in preparation for 2000m racing. As much as 80–90 per cent of an international on-water rower's training time involves moderate intensity rowing at low stroke rates (approximately 18 strokes per minute). Each session can last up to 2 hours. Regardless of whether an indoor rower is training for health or competitive performance, the majority of training time, especially during early months of training, should be directed to the development of basic endurance abilities. For new indoor rowers, these early sessions should last between 10 and 40 minutes, whereas experienced rowers should aim for sessions of between 40 and 90 minutes.

3. TRAIN AT LEAST ONCE EVERY 2 DAYS

One of the few down sides to achieving good fitness levels from regular training is that the body will quickly lose these adaptations if a similar training stimulus is not maintained. The good news is that the rate of physiological improvement is also greatest in the first weeks of training, both for new rowers and former rowers returning to training. Indoor rowers who only use the indoor rowing machine twice each week will generally struggle to achieve a steady rate of fitness gain. Likewise, an indoor rower who decides to do her weekly allocation of three training sessions on a Friday, Saturday and Sunday will experience slower gains in fitness and performance than if the same training sessions were better distributed throughout the week. Training at least once every 2 days should be a golden rule for all indoor rowers.

4. USE HIGH INTENSITY INTERVAL TRAINING SPARINGLY

High intensity interval training is an important part of preparing for indoor rowing competitions and recent research even suggests that, under certain circumstances, it may be useful for individuals with low fitness levels. In respect to indoor rowing competitions, impressive gains in 2000m race performance are achieved when a high volume/moderate intensity training programme is exclusively used, but for best results, high intensity interval sessions performed at, or above, current 2000m race capabilities are required. Training at paces that match, or slightly exceed, current 2000m racing capability provides the ideal stimulus to allow body and mind to reach peak performance. This type of training is difficult to perform well and is inevitably painful to the rower. For competitive indoor rowers the popular saying 'no pain, no gain' holds true in the final weeks before a major competition.

It is generally believed that the optimal time period for performing high intensity interval training is between four and eight weeks with no apparent performance benefit from completing more than two to three high, or very high, intensity sessions each week. This type of training places major stress on the body and increases the risk of developing injury and illness. It also becomes increasingly difficult to maintain a sufficient volume of moderate intensity base training when high intensity intervals are overused and the psychological toll of excessive interval training is substantial, especially when an indoor rower does not feel sufficiently recovered from the effects of previous training.

5. MAKE USE OF TIME TRIALS

Time trials play an important part in developing indoor rowing performance. They provide a useful opportunity to measure the cumulative effects of training and offer rowers a chance to gain confidence and experience in sustaining maximum efforts. Time trials also enable rowers to experiment with a range of pre-competition strategies including issues related to nutrition, psychological preparation and recovery from previous training. They also allow rowers to try out different pacing strategies and to develop coping strategies to help survive the toughest parts of a race. Interestingly, the benefits from the use of a time trial may be best when trial performance is disappointing. Failing

to meet performance expectations is often the best way to force a rower to reflect on what went wrong and to prepare better for the next trial.

Rowers need to approach a time trial in a similar manner to how they might approach an important competition. Trials should be planned well in advance, particularly since the weekly training load will almost certainly need to be reduced to allow sufficient recovery. Care must be taken to ensure that ongoing training objectives are not compromised by the overuse of time trials. It is also possible for an indoor rower to develop test anxiety if time trials are used too frequently. A period of about six weeks between time trials is normally enough to allow the effects of ongoing training to filter through into improved time trial performance. If necessary, time trials can be performed more frequently, possibly even once every two weeks. Under these circumstances, it is helpful to rotate the time trial distance so that the same trial distance is still not used more than once every six weeks.

The selected time trial distance should reflect the training objectives for a particular training phase. Short distances such as the 500 and 1000m trials are best used in the weeks immediately before an important 2000m event. The 1000m time trial is especially useful since it allows a good estimate of the potential 2000m performance and is likely to be less psychologically demanding. Longer distances, such as the 5000 and 10,000m trials, or even the 60 minute maximum distance row, are best suited to use in the early months of training in order to better reflect the specific training focus on base endurance. Once an indoor rower has learned how to achieve stable and successful time trial performances, the chances of good race day performance are considerably improved.

6. TAPER BEFORE IMPORTANT COMPETITIVE EVENTS

After a period of prolonged training, an indoor rower requires a period of appropriate rest and recovery to achieve peak 2000m performance. Most rowers will say they feel properly rested after 24 to 72 hours of complete rest from training. However, researchers have demonstrated that well-trained endurance athletes (including rowers) need about one to three weeks of reduced training (tapering) to achieve peak performance. Rowers who perform less than about 8–10 hours of training per week have limited opportunity to taper their training and will likely achieve peak performance after as little as 24–48 hours of rest and reduced training. On the other hand, well-trained athletes need to plan both partial (<7 days) and full tapers (7–21 days) into a training programme in order to wash out the fatigue effects that accumulate from sustained training. A partial taper requires a reduction of about 30 per cent in training volume and is suitable for use before competitions or time trials of moderate importance.

Well-trained rowers usually only perform a full taper once per season, immediately before a major competition (e.g. a national or international indoor rowing championship). Training volume is steadily reduced throughout a period of one to three weeks, until volume is approximately 40–60 per cent of pre-taper levels. During the period of tapering, it is important to maintain both the frequency and intensity of training at pre-taper levels.

Reducing training loads can be unsettling for the indoor rower used to performing high volumes of training, but it is needed to allow fine-tuning of the metabolic, cardiovascular, hormonal and especially neuromuscular systems. There may also be important benefits from tapering which improve motivation and quality of sleep. When applied correctly, tapering is associated with a typical performance improvement of about 3 per cent compared with the pre-taper performance level. This is the equivalent of around 12 seconds for an athlete with a usual 2000m performance of 7 minutes.

7. LEARN TO USE THE PERFORMANCE MONITOR TO YOUR ADVANTAGE

The popular appeal of the indoor rowing machine owes much to the development of the performance monitor. Yet, many rowers have a love-hate relationship with their digital display. It can be a great source of inspiration and motivation when the scores meet or exceed a rower's expectations. Equally, rowers can easily become distracted or overwhelmed by the large quantity and high frequency of information. The problems of distraction are made worse by the small changes in pace that are a normal part of endurance sports performance. However, unlike other endurance sports, indoor rowers have to cope with these near-instantaneous updates being placed directly in their line of sight. It takes a considerable amount of confidence and perseverance for a rower to recognise the difference between a momentary blip in pace and the true onset of physical fatigue. Even so, some of the world's very best indoor rowers have had performances ruined by the relentless and unforgiving readout of the performance monitor.

Pace fluctuations are probably influenced by small changes in an athlete's physiological sensations to ongoing exercise. Clearly, indoor rowers feel more tired at the end of a steady paced row than at the start or mid-point, but the perception of fatigue from moment to moment is more complex. Rowers often describe later sections of an even-paced row as 'easier' than earlier sections. The sensations of fatigue during exercise appear to follow a wave-like pattern rather than conventional thinking where fatigue is progressive and strictly linear. Potentially, the psychological strategies of successful indoor rowers may help attenuate the sensation of fatigue by also altering neurotransmitter release. If so, then rowers may actually be changing their physiological sensations based on their interpretation of the immediate output from the performance monitor. Until advancements in scientific research yield better information regarding real-time changes in neurobiology, indoor rowers should experiment with psychological strategies which help them to gain greater control over their subjective sensations of fatigue.

The rowing machine performance monitor can both help or hinder a rower's sense of control. The indoor rower who learns to interpret the performance monitor data carefully and respond intelligently to the onscreen information will be well placed to control their experience of indoor rowing racing and training. Helpful ways to use the performance monitor for better training and racing may include the following:

- Set an acceptable pace range in your mind around the average target pace rather than fixating on a single value (e.g. between 1:58 and 2:02 per 500m instead of simply 2:00 per 500m). If your scores drift outside the target range, just concentrate on pushing your legs a little harder, especially during the early leg drive phase of the stroke.

- During an interval workout, place a cover over the monitor on alternate intervals so that, when covered, you can only see distance remaining, relying instead on your internal sense of pacing. After the workout, compare how well you performed on the intervals where pace feedback was available versus without.

- Instead of using one screen display mode during training, try changing to a different mode after each 1000m section to reduce monotony.

- Focus on trying to hold the pace splits as stable as possible for 10- or 20-stroke sequences (but use short sequences only during challenging sessions and be willing to select different paces to better match the subjective sense of fatigue).

8. ADD PLENTY OF VARIETY TO YOUR TRAINING

Sometimes indoor rowers get stuck in a routine of using the same basic training sessions. Some individuals are even known to repeat the same basic session each day, with no alterations whatsoever. But with a little creativity and modification, even the dullest of sessions can be improved with a bit of variety. For example, adding drills to a rowing session can give the sensation that time is passing more quickly, may improve technique and need not otherwise interfere with the planned session. Other simple ideas include closing the eyes for 100 strokes while trying to develop a smoother movement; taking the feet out of the straps for 5 minutes; or just alternating between half slide and full slide rowing. These rowing-specific strategies are probably best used for less demanding training sessions or on occasions when it is hard to find the motivation to get started.

The use of running, cycling, swimming and cross-country skiing, as well as other aerobic activities, is another great way to stay motivated for indoor rowing and lowers the risk of developing an overuse injury. Many of the cardiovascular adaptations that are important for indoor rowing are also important for other aerobic-based sports. However, as a general rule, substituting indoor rowing for alternative activities on a like for like basis will not improve rowing performance once a good base of fitness is achieved. Nevertheless, the use of aerobic cross-training activities can help offset, or even prevent the loss in rowing performance which will quickly occur when the rowing specific training load is decreased.

The more difficult question to answer is whether indoor rowing performance is likely to improve when standard rowing training is supplemented by the addition of aerobic cross-training methods. Unfortunately, there is a lack of specific research to help answer this important question, but there are good reasons to expect some positive transfer of performance benefits from alterative aerobic activities, such as cycling or swimming. Certainly, Olympic rowers frequently include significant amounts of supplemental aerobic cross-training activities. Also, rowers who need to reduce body fat or body weight are likely to benefit from the additional energy cost of adding cross-training. Even team and court based sports such as soccer, tennis, squash and hockey can be useful. Indoor rowers should not be afraid to experiment with the many different ways of adding variety to specific and non-specific training activities, especially during the first months of training.

PSYCHOLOGY AND MOTIVATION FOR INDOOR ROWING

7

While many people think that exercise is boring, unpleasant and unsustainable, there are clearly plenty of indoor rowers who enjoy spending time on the rowing machine. To the uninitiated, this must sound very peculiar indeed; what could possibly be enjoyable about repeating the same movement over and over, often to the point of significant physical discomfort? When invited to answer, indoor rowers often provide a range of positive answers and sensible reasons, but they will also concede that indoor rowing can be boring, difficult and unpleasant. A major challenge to becoming a successful indoor rower is learning how to handle these contrasting experiences, both on and off the rowing machine.

There are many ways to make indoor rowing enjoyable, but it would be a mistake to think the enjoyment always comes easily. Even the most experienced rowers will have days when they don't feel any affection for rowing machines. But part of what makes them successful is their ability to cope with the tough days and to avoid throwing in the towel at the first signs of difficulty. This ability has been refined through trial and error in training, from discussions with other rowers and most of all through sustained effort. Successful indoor rowers also recognise that what worked on one occasion may not work on the next and appreciate the need for flexibility. In fact, when successful indoor rowers talk about why they enjoy rowing, they often reveal that much of their pleasure comes from finding new ways to adapt their training to improve enjoyment and performance. With these experiences in mind, this chapter contains information about the psychology of indoor rowing and provides practical suggestions to enhance motivation, enjoyment and performance during training and racing.

HOW POPULAR IS REGULAR EXERCISE?

The health benefits from regular activity are widely acknowledged and can be achieved by any adult willing to complete the weekly target of just 150 minutes of moderate intensity physical activity. This is the equivalent of just under 22 minutes per day so we would hardly be surprised if most able-bodied adults achieved these targets. Yet, survey data in the United States suggests that only 49 per cent of adults achieve these minimum recommendations, although some states fare better. For example, 60 per cent of Alaskans meet the minimum recommendations compared to only 39 per cent of Louisianans. Adults in the United Kingdom appear to struggle even more, with only 35 per cent of men and women achieving the same 150 minute weekly target. To make matters worse, these percentages are all based on official government statistics which were obtained by asking random samples of people to estimate how much activity they usually do. Using these types of self-report questionnaires introduces considerable bias, especially when the respondents are aware that they don't do as much exercise as they believe they should.

A better way to check how much exercise adults really do is to use electronic sensors worn on the body to record the number of minutes spent performing physical activity of moderate intensity or above. Using this more accurate measurement technique, only 6 per cent of men and 4 per cent of women in the United Kingdom actually achieved the minimum weekly amounts of recommended physical activity. Similar results have been revealed in other Western countries, including the United States. If most adults believe that regular exercise is important, then the low participation statistics suggest that it must be difficult to achieve in practice.

WHY DO SOME ADULTS SUCCEED AT REGULAR EXERCISE WHERE MANY OTHERS FAIL?

Typically, 50 per cent of adults drop out of exercise programmes within the first 6 months. Yet, there are clearly large numbers of adults, including many indoor rowers, who are able to adhere to regular exercise for many years despite the odds. The reasons why these individuals succeed where most others fail are complex and far from clear. Research has shown that individual personality, genetics, level of education, socio-economic status and parental influences are all important factors in a person's exercise behaviour, but these are not elements that can be easily changed. Researchers have successfully demonstrated that an individual's exercise adherence can be improved by the offer of financial incentives such as paying people to exercise or providing cash rewards when certain fitness targets are met. Exercise adherence is also improved when free gym memberships, equipment or clothing is provided, and the use of expert fitness professionals (e.g. personal trainers and motivational counsellors) also helps, but these are still very expensive and not likely to be available to most people.

An easy way to improve exercise adherence at no cost is to allow people to choose the exercise that they most enjoy. A recent scientific review highlighted that standard exercise programme features such as frequency, duration and type of exercise are particularly important determinants of adherence in groups of adults. However, men generally adhere better to vigorous intensity training, whereas women adhere better to moderate intensity training. Overall, indoor rowers will probably be more successful at regular exercise when they use an appropriate training structure that has been adjusted to suit their individual preferences, rather than when told to follow a strict daily training schedule that has been given to them without any personalisation. Accordingly, indoor rowers should think carefully before copying a generic training programme or workout plan that does not suit their individual needs.

Potentially, a better way to improve exercise adherence is to find ways to make any given training programme as enjoyable as possible for each person. What a rower thinks about during indoor rowing is one important influence on enjoyment during training and can also influence competitive performance. There are many opinions about what rowers should think about, but once again individual preferences are likely to be more important than any generic recommendation. It may take a while to develop effective thought patterns during rowing that help both enjoyment and performance, but it can help to learn about what other indoor rowers think about during their training and racing.

THINKING AND ROWING

Anyone who has spent a significant amount of time using indoor exercise equipment will already be familiar with the importance of different types of thoughts. When thoughts are positive, motivating and encouraging, the exercise time often seems to pass more quickly. On the other hand, thoughts of tiredness, discomfort and boredom can make a workout feel like it will never end. As indoor rowers gain experience of regular training, they usually gain better control over their different types of thoughts and become more capable of using particular thoughts to make training more enjoyable. It is even possible to detect consistent patterns in the way that indoor rowers apply these different thoughts during rowing.

Broadly, the thoughts experienced by indoor rowers can be usefully separated into two distinct cognitive categories known as 'association' and 'dissociation'. Rowers use association when their thoughts are task focussed and this includes thinking about the physical sensation of rowing (e.g. breathing, muscle tension). Associative thoughts can also include task-related performance information such as stroke rate, heart rate or other information commonly displayed on the rowing machine monitor (e.g. force curve, pace). In contrast, rowers use dissociation when their thoughts are unrelated to the rowing task (e.g. upcoming social events, personal relationships or when watching TV), which includes attempts to ignore the information displayed on the rowing machine performance display. Listening to music or watching a video while rowing is also a form of dissociation.

It is possible to combine associative and dissociative thoughts simultaneously, such as when a rower listens to music while also monitoring their stroke rate. Rowers can also switch quickly between different types of thoughts in sequence, but in practice, each person typically exhibits a definite preference for a particular category of thought depending on the specific influences present at that moment in time (e.g. training environment or individual motivation levels).

Researchers have tried to answer whether it is better to use associative or dissociative strategies during exercise. Unfortunately, there is no easy answer, especially since a rower's preference for the use of associative or dissociative thoughts will be influenced by features of the exercise task (e.g. intensity and duration). Additionally, the personality of an indoor rower can also influence the effectiveness of each strategy. Some rowers achieve better performances when using an associative strategy while other rowers perform better when using a dissociative strategy. Despite these complications, researchers have been able to provide a number of insights into the different cognitive strategies used by indoor rowers.

INDOOR ROWERS' PREFERENCES FOR ASSOCIATION AND DISSOCIATION

There is good evidence to show that the intensity at which indoor rowing is performed has a major influence on whether a rower will make use of associative or dissociative thoughts. Researchers at Florida State University measured the use of association and dissociation by 60 high school and university rowers (30 male and 30 female) while performing indoor rowing. The students were either experienced rowers (>three years of rowing practice) or novice rowers (<one year of rowing practice). The rowers were taught to rate their attention on a continuous scale ranging from 0 (extremely dissociative: daydreaming & external thoughts, etc.) to 10 (extremely associative: technique, breathing, etc.). Using a randomised test order, each rower completed 10 minute bouts of rowing on a Concept2 ergometer at 30, 50 and 75 per cent of maximum power and provided their attention rating at the end of each minute. After the 10 minutes, rowers also wrote what they were thinking about during rowing. This provided an additional check on each rower's focus of attention.

At the lowest exercise intensity (30 per cent of maximum power), rowers claimed to either use dissociative thoughts only or a mix of associative and dissociative thoughts. At moderate intensity (50 per cent of maximum power), rowers predominantly used a mix of associative and dissociative thoughts. When rowing at the highest intensity (75 per cent of maximum power), there was a clear preference for most rowers to make use of associative thoughts only. Interestingly, there were no systematic differences between males and females or between experienced and novice rowers. This research suggests that most indoor rowers will make extensive use of both associative and dissociative thoughts when exercising at comfortable intensities. However, once the pace of rowing reaches a level where holding a conversation becomes difficult, it appears necessary to concentrate attention more exclusively on the task of rowing. This is probably due to fact that it is hard to ignore bodily sensations when a significant amount of physical strain is present.

There is also evidence that a person's preference for associative or dissociative strategies depends on the duration of exercise. For example, marathon runners prefer to use a mix of associative and dissociative thoughts in the early part of the race before switching to predominantly dissociative thoughts in the difficult final miles. During long training sessions and indoor rowing events of an hour or more, rowers may find it helpful to try to distract themselves from the physical sensation of rowing by using dissociative thoughts, difficult though this may be.

WHEN SHOULD I USE ASSOCIATIVE OR DISSOCIATIVE THOUGHTS DURING INDOOR ROWING?

Unfortunately, there is no simple recommendation that will suit the individual needs of all rowers. Distracting dissociative type thoughts can certainly help make it seem as if time is passing more quickly. This is why different types of entertainment, such as listening to music or watching TV, are popular with indoor rowers. These methods make it easier to switch to dissociative thoughts and reduce the amount of focus directed to the task of rowing, potentially improving enjoyment and making the session feel shorter. This may be especially helpful when performing moderate intensity rowing or when completing a session of long duration.

There are also good reasons to encourage the use of associative strategies for specific occasions. Most importantly, it can be very difficult to maintain good technique when a rower is not paying close attention to their movements. Since good technique contributes to improved rowing performance, associative strategies may be better for enhancing performance. Furthermore, the use of good rowing technique is likely to reduce the risk of injury, making the use of associative thoughts directed toward effective body movements especially important for indoor rowers who have a history of indoor rowing injuries. On the other hand, it is difficult keep a narrow focus for prolonged periods.

A useful compromise to the problem of deciding what to think about during rowing is to strategically mix between associative and dissociative strategies, at least when rowing at a comfortable pace. For example, try spending 5 minutes working on a particular technique focus point (associative focus) before using the next 5 minutes to think about something unrelated to rowing or just enjoying listening to a particular song (dissociative focus). The use of 5 minute segments means that the pattern only has to be repeated a handful of times before most people will reach the end of their session. During very high intensity rowing, including 2000m racing, most coaches advise that rowers will perform better if they simply focus on their rowing and avoid external distractions. While this appears to be good advice for the majority of indoor rowers, some people may actually perform better during high intensity rowing when allowed to use distracting thoughts.

Researchers from the University of Wales in Bangor were interested to discover if personality was an important factor that influenced whether an associative or dissociative approach was more beneficial during high intensity indoor rowing. While personality is obviously very difficult to define, there do appear to be large and reliable differences between people in terms of their preference for focusing on things that are happening around them (externalisers) versus things that are happening directly to them (internalisers). Using a psychological questionnaire, the researchers were able to measure the personalities of 60 male and female sport science students according to whether they were predominantly externalisers or internalisers. Two groups were then formed; the first group containing the seven students who exhibited the strongest preferences for externalising and the second group containing the seven students who exhibited the strongest preferences for internalising. All the students were familiar with indoor rowing and completed a 15 minute time trial on the Concept2 rowing machine on two separate occasions in a randomised order. Students performed one trial while using an associative strategy and the other trial using a dissociative strategy. The associative strategy required students to focus on the performance monitor display and to read the distance completed every 15 seconds. During the dissociative strategy, students were unable to see the performance monitor and were instead asked to solve multiplication problems that were displayed on cue cards. In both conditions, students were told when they had completed 5, 10, 12 and 14 minutes of rowing to make sure that they could make reasonable pace judgments regardless of the allocated thought strategy.

The results showed that personality does influence the benefits from using associative or dissociative thoughts during high intensity indoor rowing. Students who were strong externalisers performed best when allowed to use a dissociative strategy. Conversely, students who were strong internalisers performed best when allowed to use an associative strategy (see figure 7.1). While these results suggest that individual personality differences and preferences are important considerations when deciding whether performance will be better with an associative or dissociative strategy, it is important to note that the subjects were novice rowers. Anecdotal evidence strongly suggests that associative strategies are the preferred choice of elite indoor rowers when racing over 2000m. Also, without completing psychological testing, it would be hard to know whether an indoor rower was more of an internaliser or an externaliser. A practical solution is to try these different strategies during training, paying careful attention to the intensity and duration of the task. Ultimately, personal experience may provide the clearest indication of whether an associative or dissociative strategy, or both, is most effective for use during an indoor rowing competition.

LEARNING TO IMPROVE ATTENTION DURING INDOOR ROWING

Rowers can increase the amount of time that they engage in association through regular practice. One popular strategy is to make use of a sequence

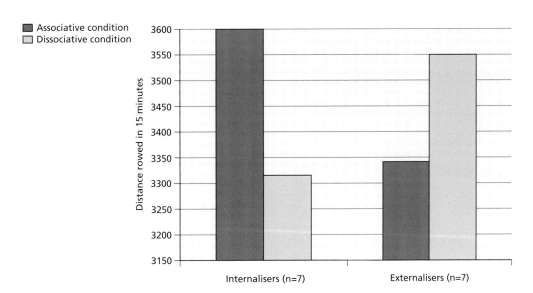

Fig 7.1 Comparison of distance rowed in 15 minutes by novice rowers according to personality and cognitive condition (Adapted from Baghurst et al. (2004))

of instructions that encourage progressive relaxation of different body segments. At first, the rower may simply think about trying to relax the fingers, hands and wrists and might even remove one hand from the handle and shake it lightly during the recovery phase. Just loosening the grip on the handle a little can help. Once the rower has detected an improvement in relaxation, usually after 10 or 20 strokes, the procedure is then repeated with the upper arms, neck, shoulders, back and all the way down to the legs. This is a great way for an indoor rower to gain an improved sense of control over their workout programme.

Progressive relaxation strategies during rowing can be very effective for developing better technique and can enhance performance by reducing the amount of unnecessary muscle activity. Inexperienced and tired rowers have a tendency to grip the oar handle tighter than necessary, wasting energy and reducing blood flow to the muscles used during rowing. This makes it harder to deliver oxygen to the active muscles and reduces the removal of carbon dioxide from the muscles, making exercise feel more difficult. The effectiveness of progressive relaxation improves considerably when regularly practised.

While associative thoughts can be helpful for preventing injury, improving technique and enhancing performance of most rowers, dissociative thoughts are still very important to successful indoor rowing training. Rowers may want to use dissociative strategies for many reasons and not necessarily because the rowing is uncomfortable or difficult. Dissociation during exercise is often a great way for people to work through personal or professional problems or just to engage in a spot of daydreaming to help pass the time. Depending on the objectives of the training session, it may be appropriate to use dissociative thoughts only, or to alternate between associative and dissociative strategies. Hopefully, you will be able to apply this information to suit your individual circumstances. It is important to be flexible in your approach and to experiment with different types of thoughts according to personal preference. Where possible, try to plan your use of associative and dissociative thoughts before beginning a session. This will make it easier to evaluate what works better according to different circumstances and to improve your ability to predict suitable strategies for increasing future indoor rowing performance and enjoyment.

TAKING CONTROL OF YOUR ROWING

One of the most frustrating experiences that can happen to an indoor rower is failing to complete a training session or race as planned. In the worst case, the rower will abandon the rowing machine altogether, often saying that it wasn't worth continuing when the pace was slower than the target demanded. There are various reasons for these failures including unrealistic initial expectations, loss of self-belief or simply a loss of focus. To reduce the risk of failure, indoor rowers need to feel in control of their rowing. In fact, much of the way that an experienced coach prepares an athlete for success is through teaching them how to set targets appropriately in order to improve their confidence and sense of control. Nothing will challenge a rower's sense of control more than the physical stress of a hard workout. The solution is to identify sensible exercise targets and experiment with a variety of psychological strategies that provide experience in developing control and self-belief.

SETTING GOALS

A useful way to help take control of indoor rowing training and racing is to set clear goals. In the first instance, it is worth writing down short- and long-term goals for what you want to achieve from your indoor rowing. These goals can be performance focussed (e.g. rowing 2000m in under 9 minutes), process focussed (e.g. rowing with good technique for 30 minutes) during a particular session) or outcome focussed (e.g. improving muscle tone). For each goal that you set, you will need to decide if it is likely to be achieved quickly (short-term goals) or something that will take much longer to achieve, possibly requiring months or even years to achieve (long-term goals). Keep in mind that many people find it difficult to sustain regular exercise for more than 6 months, so consider restricting your initial long-term goals to this length of time.

Indoor rowers often dismiss the importance of actually writing their goals on paper. Yet, this simple act is very important since it encourages a person to separate their reasons for training into separate components rather than a hazy, general idea. The more carefully you specify each goal the better the chance of achieving it, especially if the goal is measurable in some way. The original intention of broad, non-specific goals is easy to misrepresent at a later stage, especially if progress has been disappointing. It will help to state a weight loss goal in terms of losing a specific amount of weight within a defined period of rowing training rather than just deciding to lose any amount of weight. For example, a weight loss target could be written as, 'Reduce bodyweight

---

Examples of short-term goals

- Row continuously for 15 minutes
- Row for 60 minutes at conversational pace but take a 10 minute break to stretch and drink after 40 minutes
- Try to make a technique improvement for 500m after every 5 minutes of rowing
- Keep the stroke rate between 18 and 20 strokes per minute for the first 20 minutes of rowing
- Complete FOUR rowing sessions this week
- Try the progressive relaxation technique during any 10 minute section of today's workout

Examples of long-term goals

- Reduce 2000m time from 08:40 to 08:25 in 6 weeks
- Row 1000km in 6 months
- Increase VO_2max by 10% in 10 weeks
- Complete the national indoor rowing marathon after 5 months of training
- Increase from 3 training sessions per week to 5 sessions per week within 3 months
- Complete a 10km time trial after every 8 weeks of training

Fig 7.2 Examples of short- and long-term goals

from 75.0 to 72.5kg within eight weeks by completing 2000kcal of rowing each week'. Table 7.1 lists a number of clearly stated short-term and long-term goals that will help you to develop better wording for your own goals.

At this point, having some understanding of what is realistically possible for a given ability and amount of training time is important to consider. For many indoor rowers, this will require expert advice or careful consideration of information available in books and magazines. Even just talking to other indoor rowers can be informative and helpful to establishing suitable goals.

GETTING STARTED

It is often difficult for both experienced and inexperienced indoor rowers to begin their first indoor rowing session after a long period of inactivity. There is a very reasonable concern that the first few minutes of rowing will be uncomfortable on the body and the display scores disappointingly poor. However, there is no point in worrying about these first minutes. Instead of starting out with ambitious hopes, it is usually best to set a simple target for the first session. Rather than focusing on exercise intensity, set a basic target for the volume of training to perform in this first session. Inexperienced rowers should pick a set amount of time (e.g. 15 minutes) as their initial volume, whereas more experienced indoor rowers can set their volume according to either time or distance. Something in the order of 10–30 minutes is a good starting volume regardless of previous experience. Just focus on completing the session no matter how slow the pace needs to be. Repeat the same session every few days until it starts to feel easy enough to slowly start to add a bit more volume. The pace will probably quicken over time without conscious effort but concentrate on staying comfortable and just adding a little more volume when possible. There is no need to rush during these first sessions. One benefit to starting from a low fitness level is that the improvements in exercise capacity occur relatively quickly and are easy to notice. By taking a steady approach to these first sessions, it is much easier to build confidence and develop a suitable routine.

Here are several key points to keep in mind when beginning your training:

- Before starting a session, make sure to specify a realistic volume (time or distance as appropriate to your experience) to complete.
- Try to use long effective strokes at a low stroke rate (e.g. 20 strokes per minute) rather than short ineffective strokes at a high stroke rate (e.g. 28 stroke per minute).
- Especially on days when you are feeling good, don't do any more than you planned.
- Don't focus too much on the performance monitor, just make occasional checks to keep check of your overall progress.
- Row at an intensity which would allow you to have a conversation but not to be able to sing.
- Focus on staying relaxed and making sure rowing is enjoyable during the first 5 minutes of a session.
- Buy a seat pad or just sit on a soft towel if you find the seat uncomfortable.
- Listen to music or watch a video.

- Focus on maintaining a consistent stroke-to-stroke performance for short sections of 20 strokes each.
- Consider purchasing a heart rate monitor to help keep you in a healthy training zone.
- Try to get a friend to train with you on a regular basis.

Ten habits of highly effective indoor rowers

1. Keeping a written diary or online training log of all training sessions
2. Avoiding the temptation of doing too much in a single training session
3. Training with a partner or group of friends
4. Developing a structured approach to both nutrition and training
5. Finding creative ways to add variety to indoor rowing sessions
6. Including a time trial or other fitness measurement once every six weeks to track progress
7. Modifying rather than scrapping a training session when unforeseen difficulties occur (e.g. injury, illness or lack of time)
8. Supplementing indoor rowing sessions with regular cross-training activities (e.g. resistance training, running, spinning classes)
9. Making rowing technique improvement a regular focus of training
10. Developing a range of associative and dissociative cognitive strategies to suit the demands of different training sessions

ADDING VARIETY AND ENJOYMENT DURING INDOOR ROWING

The following ideas and strategies can be used to add variety to indoor rowing training.

SOCIAL ROWING

A great way to make indoor rowing more enjoyable is to exercise with other people. Some fitness centres and gyms now offer 'crew classes' where an instructor takes a group of indoor rowers through a variety of rowing-specific workouts. These classes are usually great fun and can be a good way to meet new people and pick up some technical pointers.

Research also provides strong support for the benefits of working out with other people. In fact, exercising with a partner, or as part of a group, is one of the best ways to improve adherence. It's much harder to skip a training session if you know that someone is waiting at the gym for you to arrive. Interestingly, the benefits from training with a partner appear to be even greater for women than men, especially in the first months of training.

PACE PLAY

One of the great advantages of most indoor rowing equipment is that work rates are easy to adjust. Treadmills, bikes and cross-trainers have a certain nuisance factor that comes from having to adjust buttons or knobs and often discourages users from changing pace. There can be benefits to varying pace during a training session, especially for indoor rowers who learn to make good use of their internal sense of pacing. The freedom to alter exercise intensity allows the exerciser a greater sense of control and can even reduce the physiological strain of exercise.

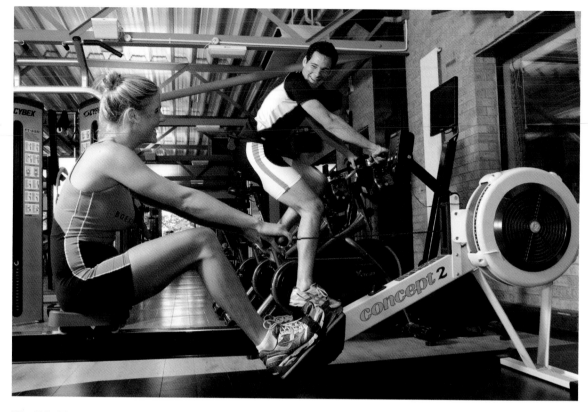

Fig 7.3 Training with a friend or partner substantially increases exercise adherence

Researchers in New Zealand monitored the physiological responses of recreational gym users during 5000m sub-maximal efforts on a Concept2 rowing machine. The subjects in this study first learned how to use a perceived exertion scale which ranged from 6 (no exertion) to 20 (maximal exertion). On one 5000m trial, the subjects were told to select the intensity of rowing that corresponded to an exertion score of 15 (hard) but were unable to see any information from the performance monitor about how hard they were actually working. This focussed the subjects on using their own sense of pace judgement and made it easier to alter their pace at any point in the 5000m row.

On a separate day, the subjects completed another 5000m row but this time they were able to see the power output on the performance monitor and the researchers instructed each subject to row at a particular power output. Unknown to the subjects, these power outputs were the average power outputs that each subject achieved during the first trial when they could not see any pace information.

The power produced during each stroke was unsurprisingly more variable during the self-paced trial than when subjects could see the performance monitor. However, body temperature, muscle activity and blood lactate levels were all lower in the self-paced trial. When subjects were asked afterwards about which trial they found more difficult, most subjects found the constant pace trial harder than the self-paced trial. Further research with experienced rowers is still needed, but this study suggests that indoor rowers may be able to reduce the physiological and psychological strain of a training session by focussing on how rowing actually feels and making minor changes in pace rather than focussing on rowing at one steady pace for the entire duration.

ADDING STRUCTURE TO THE SESSIONS

During a training session, adjust the performance monitor to display the power per stroke. Try counting how many strokes you can achieve in 2 minutes while keeping the pace within a narrow range. Good rowers can usually row with less than 2.5 per cent variation in their power per stroke for an unbroken sequence of 20 strokes or more (e.g. at a power output of 200W, good rowers can keep within 195–205W). Most beginner rowers can usually row with less than 5 per cent variation in their power per stroke.

Plan small pace changes at regular intervals to reduce the monotony of fixed pace training. This strategy can often make it feel like time is passing quicker than fixed pace rowing. However, make sure the pace changes are small enough to allow a speedy return to the standard training pace, for example:

- 6 minutes at usual pace (e.g. 2:05/500m) then 4 minutes at a slightly faster pace (e.g. 2:02/500m)
- 40 seconds at usual pace (e.g. 2:05/500m) then 20 seconds at a slightly faster pace (e.g. 2:02/500m)

DAYDREAMING

Daydreaming is a great way for most people to escape from the monotony of repetitive tasks. It is easy enough to escape the slow class, dull meeting or routine housework with this type of unstructured mental activity. During indoor rowing, it is usually harder to sustain a daydreaming episode but with a little practice it becomes much easier. Start the session by developing a steady rhythm and easy pace for about 5 or 10 minutes of rowing before allowing your mind to drift away. This will be hard to do if you are exercising in a busy gym. In this case, try closing your eyes and eliminate the external environment as much as possible. Playing familiar music through headphones is helpful for daydreaming too, but commercial radio stations often have annoying disruptions which can break concentration. If you are rowing in a quiet location, try staring into space. Fix your gaze on an object or section of wall in front of you and try to keep your eyes there for twenty strokes. As you stare, you may find that the simple act of counting strokes helps move your thoughts toward an enjoyable daydreaming.

It is best to avoid unstructured daydreaming if you need to focus on improving stroke technique since this would be an unhelpful distraction from technique improvements. However, you could try imagining yourself making a specific technical change. A good way to do this is to create an imaginary live video stream of you rowing. Select one technique point that you want to change and then imagine yourself rowing with this new technique. Try this for 10 strokes then move your imaginary camera to a new position. Be creative with your footage; don't just go for the standard broadcast-type angles from the side or front of the machine. Instead, move the camera to interesting and unusual positions, such as directly above, as if you were sitting on the ceiling having an out-of-body experience! It's a fun way to practise visualisation and improve your stroke technique. If you have a video camera, you could even take this one step further by hooking a live feed of your rowing to a TV and watching yourself rowing in real time. This is actually something that is popular with Olympic rowing teams during indoor practices for exactly the same reasons.

KEYWORDS

Repeating a keyword at the end of each drive phase can help rowers maintain focus, especially during tough sections of a workout. Select a keyword with a positive meaning or that encourages good technique and form. Repeat the same word, either internally or externally, for a sequence of approximately 10 strokes. Examples of possible keywords to try include:

- Strong
- Focus
- Good
- Control
- Long strokes
- Sit up
- Persistence
- Relentless

When selected with care, keywords can really help focus the mind and body in specific ways that can help make rowing better. Another helpful reminder may come from investing in several motivational posters to put up in your training room, especially if they contain good key words.

COUNTING STROKES

While counting sheep might help people get to sleep, counting strokes during rowing definitely won't. In fact, counting strokes is possibly the most popular way to help break long periods of rowing into shorter, more manageable sections. This strategy is helpful during racing or training and is often used by Olympic rowers during training. It's also true that many coxes use this strategy when trying to keep on-water rowers focussed. A good number to try might be 100 since at a typical rating of 20 strokes per minute, 5 minutes is required to count-up and 5 minutes to count-down, resulting in 10 minutes of rowing without any need to check the performance monitor.

EYES CLOSED ROWING

Another good way to remove focus away from the performance monitor is to just close your eyes. This works even better when you combine it with stroke counting or mental imaging. You may even find that your average pace gets better when rowing with eyes closed. Some indoor rowers become too dependent on the performance monitor and end up staying at a safe training pace when they may work better by allowing pace to fluctuate according to preferred exertion.

TAKE A BREAK DURING A SESSION

Indoor rowers often think that it is better to row continuously for 40 minutes than to complete two sets of 20 minutes at the same average pace with a short break between sets. However, the adaptations to endurance training appear to be similar. In fact, it might even be better to break a long training session into shorter sections since this allows a chance to stretch, drink and freshen up. The risk of developing an injury can also be reduced by taking short breaks during long training sessions.

SHORTEN THE SESSION

If you occasionally find yourself caught short for available training time, then consider doing a short workout but at a higher pace. The health and performance benefits from short lasting, intense rowing (e.g. 20 minutes at 90 per cent of maximum heart rate) are actually very similar to those gained from long sessions of moderate intensity rowing (e.g. 60 minutes at 70 per cent of maximum heart rate). This may seem counterintuitive, but scientific research is now providing strong support for the use of short, intense training sessions and it may be better to complete a short session at any pace than to skip training altogether. Just be careful that you don't disrupt your regular training with too much use of shortened sessions. This is particularly important if weight loss is a major goal of your training, since the number of kcals expended will decrease in proportion to reduction in distance rowed. If weight loss is one of your goals and you find that you need to use a shorter session than planned, then try eating less food for that day. The calorie counter on the performance monitor can be used to identify how much less energy should be eaten. For example, if your usual training session requires 700kcal and the shortened session requires only 400kcal, then see if you can find sensible ways to eliminate 300kcal from your food intake that day (e.g. six chicken nuggets, whole milk latte (standard size), half of a French bread cheese pizza).

High intensity training is suitable for rowers with good health and can be suitable for individuals with specific health conditions when approved by a physician or GP. Be sure to start with at least 5 minutes of warm-up exercises before starting high intensity training and it is wise to complete a 5 minute cool down afterwards, especially for rowers aged 40 or older. Examples of short, high intensity sessions that can be used as a convenient alternative to standard training include:

- 5 minute warm-up, rowing – 30 seconds at 2000m race pace with 30 seconds recovery for a total of 15 minutes – 5 minute cool down, rowing
- 5 minute warm-up, rowing – 20 strokes at a rate of 28–34 strokes per minute followed by 20 strokes of easy rowing; repeat for a total of 15 minutes – 5 minute cool down, rowing
- 5 minute warm-up, rowing – 60 seconds of maximum pressure rowing but at a rate of only 20 strokes per minute, then immediately increase the stroke rate by 2 strokes per minute, repeating the maximum pressure for another 60 seconds; continue to increase the stroke rate by 2 strokes per minute until a stroke rate of 30 has been completed; row gently for 3 minutes before repeating the series once more – end with a 5 minute cool down, rowing.

CHANGE THE DISPLAY SETTINGS

Many indoor rowers use the same display screen every time they train. It can be reassuring to see a familiar pace or power output. However, it is easy to become overly attached to one specific number and this can create difficulties on days when the number is difficult to maintain. For example, if you have had a week off training due to illness, then it may be distracting to see numbers that don't match your normal expectations. You could simply flip the performance monitor out of sight, but an alternative is to use an unfamiliar screen setting. For indoor rowers who are used to watching the pace per 500m screen, simply switching over to the power output screen for a while can be helpful.

RACING SIMULATION

Indoor rowers who enjoy competing may enjoy some race simulation practice in training. This involves imagining that they are in a real race, either on-water or in the indoor rowing arena. It helps to have a sequence of imagined distance markers which correspond to the distance remaining on the ergometer display. For example, if you have familiarity with a stretch of river with known distance markers, then try closing your eyes and imagining yourself racing down this same stretch of water, noting the key features which correspond to actual distances such as bridges, boathouses, trees or other riverbank features. An alternative is to imagine that you are running laps of a 400m track. The straights and bends of a standard running track are all 100m in length. Indoor rowers often find this imaging approach works best toward the end of a session, such as the last 10 or 20 minutes. There is even computer software which removes the need to imagine an on-water race by using the pace information from a connected rowing machine to

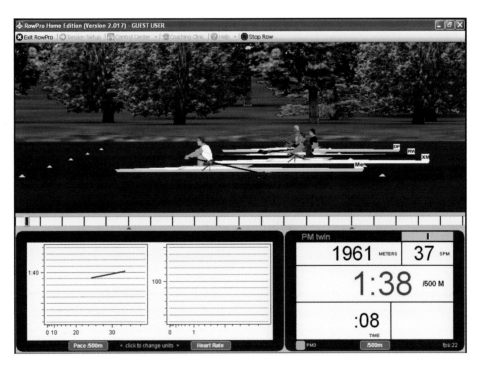

Fig 7.4 Screenshot from the RowPro software for use with the Concept2 indoor rowing machine

propel an on-screen boat against other competitors in a simulated race (see figure 7.4).

TRY A LITTLE TECHNOLOGY

In the near future, there is the very exciting prospect that technology will enable indoor rowers to select from a range of virtual rowing environments. Imagine sitting down on your machine and putting on 3D video glasses and surround sound headphones. You scroll through a list of possible options including a rural section of the Danube at dawn, complete with wildlife, or a tourist's view of Paris in summer, as viewed from the clear waters of the Seine; or how about a dusky autumn evening row past Boathouse Row in Philadelphia? The motion sensing technology incorporated into the headset could allow a full 360-degree view while noise-cancelling headphones could substitute the drone of a rowing machine for the tranquil sounds of river and oars. At present, this sort of system is not commercially available for rowing, but similar ideas are already available for indoor cycling, running and cross-country skiing using videos from picturesque locations. Without doubt, something suitable for indoor rowing will be available very soon.

MUSIC

Listening to music during indoor rowing is clearly very popular. In fact, some indoor rowers say they would prefer to skip training altogether if they didn't have their usual music playlist available. While there is a popular perception that music enhances exercise performance, research does not always support this view and it is likely that individual preference has a strong influence in determining if music will be helpful. When music has been shown to improve exercise performance,

researchers have usually suggested the following possible explanations:

- Reduction in the perception of fatigue
- Improved relaxation
- Increased muscle coordination and synchro-nisation
- Increase in arousal and improved mood levels

The effect of music on indoor rowing performance has interested various researchers. In one study, Hungarian researchers examined the effect of fast- and slow-paced music on indoor rowing sprint performance. Twenty-two trained rowers (male and female) each completed three separate 500m sprints on a Concept2 machine while listening to either no music, slow music or fast music during each of the 500m sprints. Extracts of classical music from Beethoven's Symphony Number 7 in A major were taken from the second (allegretto; 72 beats per minute) and final movements (allegro con brio; 144 beats per minute) to provide the slow and fast music, respectively. The researchers randomised the order in which the different music conditions were played to rowers to avoid any confounding effects due to fatigue. Average 500m performance was 107.4 seconds when no music was played but was significantly faster when either slow music was played (106.8 seconds) or when fast music was played (105.3 seconds). During the fast-paced music, the average stroke rate of the rowers increased from 33 strokes per minute (no music) to 35 strokes per minute.

In another study, this time with novice male and female university rowers, 40 minute indoor rowing performance on a Concept2 machine was recorded once per week for 10 weeks (i.e. 10 rowing sessions). The rowers were instructed to cover as much distance as possible in the 40 minutes and were able to see their pace, stroke rate, elapsed time and distance completed on the performance monitor. Once each rower achieved a stable week-to-week 40 minute distance (baseline phase), they were randomly allocated to only one of the following interventions:

- A pop music soundtrack of chart hits (dissociative condition)
- Video of the world rowing championships (dissociative condition)
- Soundtrack of a cox providing semi-frequent instructions to focus on specific aspects of rowing (associative condition)

Each rower continued to perform the weekly 40-minute maximal rows until they had completed the remainder of the 10 original sessions, but now did so using the intervention to which they were allocated (intervention phase). The average 40 minute distance completed during the intervention phase was compared to the average 40 minute distance during the baseline phase. The three rowers who listened to the coxing soundtrack improved their performance by 3.8 per cent, the three rowers who watched the video improved by 1.3 per cent while the three rowers who listened to music improved by 0.8 per cent. However, these results must be interpreted with caution due to the small sample of rowers in each intervention. Also, the rowers were not allowed to choose their own music. Nevertheless, this study does suggest that listening to music during indoor rowing training can be helpful, although other strategies such as watching a motivational video may be better.

The use of music during indoor rowing, whether for training, racing or both, is probably a decision best left to each individual. For indoor rowers who do wish to listen to music, it is a good idea to experiment with different types and speeds of music. It may even be helpful to trial different ways of playing the music, either by listening through headphones or using speakers. Lastly, if rowers are planning to compete in an indoor rowing event without the assistance of music, then it is sensible to perform at least some training without any music.

WATCHING TELEVISION

Many indoor rowers make use of their indoor rowing session to catch up on a favourite TV series, watch an interesting documentary or just keep an eye on the latest news. The increased availability of large screen TVs, video projectors and the portability of laptop computers provides most rowers with the option of watching something that can be both visually stimulating and entertaining.

In the past, indoor rowers discovered that the noise from their rowing often drowned out the sound of the TV. However, the latest rowing machines are considerably quieter and wireless headsets can be purchased if required. The ability to simultaneously row and engage in TV viewing at the same time does offer indoor rowers an excellent incentive to train, however, it is best used during moderate or easy training sessions only. During harder intensity sessions, it is difficult to listen to dialogue or keep track of a complex storyline. In these situations, watching TV while rowing is likely to be very annoying. Save the TV viewing for recovery sessions or for days when you are feeling low on motivation and just need a bit of visual inspiration. That said, it is still better to watch TV from the indoor rower than from the couch!

LISTEN TO A PODCAST OR AN AUDIO BOOK

Audio books and podcasts are also good to help pass time on the rowing machine. As with TV viewing, the extent to which this is a good method of entertainment will depend on a person's ability to concentrate on rowing and thinking at the same time. If the session intensity remains relatively easy or moderate, then it should be fine, but if the purpose of the rowing session is to improve fitness, then it might be best to save these more cognitively demanding forms of entertainment for another day.

MOTIVATIONAL SOUNDTRACKS

Some indoor rowers enjoy listening to a motivational soundtrack during training. On-water rowers have even been known to record the audio commentary from a cox to listen to during indoor rowing. One company even sells software for use with indoor rowing machines that provides motivational audio from a cox linked to the performance information displayed on the monitor. The cox's calls are matched to the distance remaining in the workout and can be mixed with music. It is even possible to set the speed of the music to match the rowing pace and section of the workout, playing faster music as the finish line approaches. This is certainly an appealing way to make training and racing more interesting.

TRY A DIFFERENT WORKOUT ENVIRONMENT

The workout environment is also an important consideration for enjoyment of indoor rowing. Most rowing machines are easy to move which makes it relatively easy to make indoor rowing an outdoor activity. It is worth noting that endurance capacity is best when exercising in temperatures of approximately 10°C and slightly reduced at a typical room temperature of 20°C. Taking your rowing machine outdoors, especially to a cooler environment, may actually boost your performance and provide a welcome change of scenery.

INDOOR ROWING FOR ON-WATER ROWERS

8

Indoor rowing is an essential part of preparation for on-water rowing competitions. Rowing machines offer an acceptable method for testing the fitness of individual oarsmen and oarswomen and provide coaches with quantitative data to help make crew selections. Most on-water training programmes include plenty of indoor rowing, especially during the preparation phase of the season and when bad weather restricts boat-based training. It may seem unremarkable that on-water rowers make extensive use of indoor rowing machines, but this is a relatively recent phenomenon.

INDOOR ROWING MACHINES
THE RISE OF THE MACHINES

Indoor rowing machines were a rare sight in rowing clubs prior to the 1980s. Some rowers were using ergometers such as the Gamut and Gjessing for training, testing and research projects, but most on-water rowers had little or no access to rowing machines. Instead, on-water rowers and rowing clubs usually spent their equipment budgets on boats, oars and basic gym equipment. Even when rowing machines were purchased, the small numbers supplied rarely offered a practical training alternative for large teams. Instead, most competitive on-water rowers performed supplemental training in rowing tanks or used cross-training activities such as running or cycling. When fitness tests were considered necessary, non-specific assessment methods were used (e.g. pull-ups, 1 mile run) and crew selection procedures were heavily weighted toward on-water seat racing and the subjective opinions of the coach. It was only in the years after Concept2 rowing machines entered the market that a major shift in sporting culture occurred.

Production of the Model A rowing ergometer, Concept2's first rowing machine, started in 1981. However, it was only after the Model B was introduced in 1984 that on-water rowers everywhere started to take indoor rowing machines seriously. The growing consensus among competitive rowers was that this second generation of Concept2 machines provided a good simulation of on-water rowing. An important feature introduced with the Model B was a sophisticated performance monitor that was able to deliver very accurate measurements of rowing power, making it possible to display an equivalent boat speed and to measure the time to complete a set distance (e.g. 2000m or 2500m).

The overwhelming popularity of Concept2's machines with on-water rowers is probably best explained by its affordability. Although Concept2 machines are now widely used by anyone, the original intention of the designers was to build a machine that was acceptable and affordable to individual rowers. The comparatively low cost of Concept2 machines attracted much interest from on-water rowers. Individual Model B machines were shipped to the homes of many on-water rowers, while large orders of Model B rowing machines were delivered to rowing clubs, universities and national rowing federations. The demand for Concept2 machines grew exponentially and although new models were introduced in later years, the basic design and performance monitor features have remained. Within a decade, a simple idea that started as an upturned bicycle nailed to the floor of a Vermont dairy barn had transformed a sport which hadn't experienced such seismic shifts in widespread practice since the introduction of the sliding seat some 100 years earlier.

BENEFITS OF ROWING MACHINE FOR ALL ABILITIES

It is now standard practice to begin the training of new on-water rowers with a session on the indoor rowing machine. It's much easier to teach the basic sequence of movements using a rowing machine than it is a boat, and this order of events surely enhances the rate of on-water skill learning as well as making for a safer and more enjoyable experience. At the other extreme of competitive ability, elite rowers have accepted the importance of rowing machines as an essential part of training and individual performance monitoring. In particular, all candidates seeking selection to

their national team are well aware of the need to achieve a specific level of indoor rowing machine performance before they can expect their attempts to be taken seriously by selectors. There is no other Olympic sport that depends more on a piece of fitness equipment which is a common sight in homes and gyms everywhere. Across all levels of ability, indoor rowing machines have become an essential feature of on-water rowing.

ROWING MACHINE DESIGN AND ON-WATER ROWING

It is a remarkable fact that the basic Concept2 machine design has changed very little in over 30 years and yet remains the most popular brand with on-water rowers. However, the recent efforts of manufacturers, including Concept2, to both revise the basic ergometer design and to add innovative accessories to improve the simulation of on-water rowing suggest that there is plenty of opportunity for improvement. Possibly the main driver for progress is the need to better reflect the skill demands of on-water rowing, something which has been a lingering criticism of many on-water rowers.

In the next sections, we will consider the value of indoor rowing machines for on-water rowing and consider how design modifications can improve the skill demands and sensation of on-water rowing. We will also compare the physiological responses during indoor and on-water rowing to provide a better indication of the validity of using indoor rowing machines for training and testing. The value of using indoor rowing machines to help inform crew selection procedures is also discussed.

REPLICATING THE DYNAMICS OF ON-WATER ROWING

There are two rowing machine designs that have gained popularity with on-water rowers; the straight pull design and the circular pull design.

STRAIGHT PULL MODELS

Straight pull models such as the Concept2, Rowperfect and WaterRower use a single handle connected to a chain or rope that can be pulled in a straight line. Each machine uses a handle return mechanism which provides a small amount of recoil force and removes the need for the user to actively return the handle to the catch position as would be necessary during on-water rowing. The patterns of handle excursion are also different to on-water rowing. Most modern straight pull rowing machines allow some freedom for handle movement in any direction, but this hardly compensates for the basic fact that these machines cannot simulate the essential handle trajectories used during on-water rowing. Consequently, substantial differences exist between on-water and indoor rowing with respect to arm, shoulder and trunk movements, and to a lesser degree, lower body movements. Straight pull rowing machines provide a better approximation of the body movements used during sculling than sweep oar rowing but the basic design of a straight pull machine will always be a major barrier to simulating on-water rowing. If on-water rowers are truly seeking a rowing machine to maximise the benefits of indoor rowing for the purposes of on-water training and crew selection, especially for sweep oared rowing, then they will have to make the difficult switch away from the highly popular straight pull design to the more representative and suitable circular pull machine design.

CIRCULAR PULL MODELS

Circular pull machines are far better suited than straight pull machines for improving the transfer of physiological adaptations from indoor rowing to on-water rowing. They also provide a significant improvement in the validity of using rowing machines for on-water selection procedures. Extensive scientific tests are not required to support these most basic of observations. Yet, the limitations of straight pull rowing machines do not appear to be a major concern of contemporary on-water rowers, coaches and national team selectors. The dominance of straight pull rowing machines over circular pull machines is quite possibly a quirk of modern rowing that earlier generations of rowing experts would not have predicted.

Historically, it was the circular pull design that was the popular choice of on-water rowers, even though the numbers produced were very small. For example, the Narragansett indoor rowing machine was one such circular pull device that gained popularity during the early part of the 20th century, especially with the predominantly sweep based college rowing teams in North America. Since then, there have been limited efforts to mass-produce a circular pull machine, but it is likely that this situation will change within the next decades as on-water rowers look for a 'new' way to gain competitive advantage.

Recently, the Australian company Oartec have produced their 'Rowing Simulator' which has a circular-pull motion and uses an air-braked resistance system, similar to Concept2 and Rowperfect machines. Since its introduction in 2007, the Oartec Simulator has attracted interest from on-water rowers and coaches despite its higher cost when compared to the straight pull machines that populate most rowing clubs. The Simulator can be configured for either a sculling or a sweep configuration and the handles can be adjusted to match the horizontal and vertical trajectory of real oars. It is even possible to rotate the oar handles in a feathering motion. These features help make the Oartec Simulator feel much closer to actual rowing than most other rowing machines.

There are good reasons to think that circular pull machines may grow in popularity with competitive rowers who want to enhance the transfer of technical and physiological gains made during a period of land based to on-water rowing. Nevertheless, the current levels of investment in straight pull machines will make it very difficult for circular pull machines to recapture the market for on-water rowers. Two interesting products worth mentioning are the Row-Right Sculling Simulator (www.row-right.com) and the Swingulator (www.rowinginnovations.com), these products make it possible to use a circular pulling pattern by modifying a standard Concept2 machine. Altering the configuration of a rowing machine is likely to prove far easier than changing the current on-water rowing culture where straight pull machines are clearly dominant.

SLIDING ERGOMETERS

One way that rowing machine manufacturers have attempted to enhance the simulation of on-water rowing is to use a sliding foot stretcher in addition to a sliding seat. Although the idea of mounting a rowing machine on wheels was not new, it was only after the Rowperfect machine was developed in 1988 that many on-water rowers became familiar with the benefits of a freely mobile foot

stretcher. Several years later, Concept2 introduced slides that allowed Model C, D or E machines to be mounted on sliding rails (see figure 8.1) and have recently launched the Dynamic Indoor Rower. The Rowperfect and Concept2 slides allow multiple machines to be physically connected together, enabling each rower to feel the forces applied by other rowers. The use of connected rowing machines by an entire crew may help improve on-water synchronization, especially in crew sculling. At present, there are no plans to use either the Dynamic Indoor Rower or sliders at the Crash B Indoor Rowing Championships.

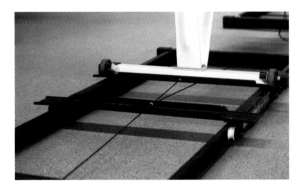

Fig 8.1 Sliders for use with the Concept2 indoor rowing machines

When using a stationary indoor rowing machine, the rower has to move almost all of their body weight back and forward during each stroke while the machine stays still. But, during on-water rowing, it is actually the lighter mass of the boat (~17 kg for a single scull and oars) that is pulled toward the rower, which requires less energy. By either mounting the rowing machine on slides or allowing the combined foot stretcher and flywheel unit to move freely, the lighter mass of the machine (~17 to 26 kg depending on machine model) does most of the moving while the heavier mass of the rower remains relatively stationary.

Compared with stationary machines, these sliding ergometers should provide energy savings, alter physiological adaptations and potentially decrease the risk of injury by reducing the compression force on joints. Many experienced on-water rowers will also testify that sliding ergometers provide a more realistic feeling of actual rowing than stationary ergometer rowing. Nevertheless, competitive rowing programmes have generally been slow to adopt sliding ergometers in large numbers, possibly suggesting that the perceived benefits are insufficient to warrant the extra financial cost. However, it is probably also the case that the uptake of sliding ergometers is influenced by the national team testing requirements in various countries. For example, in the United Kingdom, all national team athletes are expected to use a stationary Concept2 machine, whereas in Australia, national team athletes are now expected to use a Concept2 machine mounted on slides. Over time, it is conceivable that more clubs in Australia will increase their purchases of sliders to copy the national team testing strategy, and in doing so, rowers in Australian clubs are more likely to gain the benefits of slide-based indoor rowing.

WHAT PHYSIOLOGICAL AND BIOMECHANICAL DIFFERENCES ARE THERE BETWEEN STATIONARY AND SLIDING ROWING MACHINES?

The biomechanical and physiological responses to rowing on sliding and stationary ergometers have been compared in a number of scientific investigations. For example, researchers in Denmark examined the responses of seven female national team rowers during rowing on either a stationary or slide mounted Concept2 machine. Physiological and biomechanical measures were obtained during a maximal 6 minute effort as well as during sub-maximal rowing at equal power outputs (approximately 40 per cent, 55 per cent and 70 per cent of maximum pace). Key measures included heart rate, oxygen consumption and biomechanical measures such as stroke length and peak force that were obtained from handle force and position measuring devices.

The physiological measurements were reasonably similar between the sliding and stationary conditions. For example, heart rate and oxygen consumption did not differ between the two conditions for either sub-maximal or maximal rowing. However, there were differences in other measures. For example, neuromuscular activity of the legs was reduced during the late recovery and early drive phases when using the sliding ergometer. The rowers also used slightly higher stroke rates when rowing on the sliding ergometer (typically one to three strokes per minute higher at each power output), and stroke lengths during maximal rowing were slightly shorter in the stationary versus the sliding condition (by an average of 3cm) but similar during sub-maximal rowing.

FORCE AND POSITION SENSORS

Rowing machines can be fitted with force and position sensors to give qualitative and quantitative technique information and feedback. Handle force can be obtained using a force transducer connected between the handle and drive chain, while handle position can be measured using a rotary potentiometer or optical encoder. By integrating handle force and position data, a force-distance curve can be generated. These curves are specific to each rower and reflect their unique sequence of body movements and muscle activity. Stylistic features of a rower's on-water force curve are often reflected in their ergometer force curve, suggesting that patterns of force application are reasonably similar between indoor and on-water rowing. The shape of this curve provides a coach with useful information about each rower's technique. For example, rowers who increase their emphasis on leg drive typically increase the steepness of their force curve and reach peak force sooner. It is also likely that performance in some on-water rowing events (e.g. quadruple sculls) can be improved if all crew members reach peak force at a similar drive position and time. While it would be better to make these measurements during actual rowing, a reasonable indication can be obtained from the use of an instrumented rowing machine.

Better evidence to support the value of taking force measurements during indoor rowing for predicting on-water rowing is available. In a study conducted at the University of Sydney, rowers of different ability levels completed a maximal 6 minute test on an instrumented rowing machine, making it possible to examine how similar each rower's force curve was between separate drive phases (stroke-to-stroke consistency). On average, force curve consistency was highest in elite oarsmen (95 per cent similarity) in comparison with club level oarsmen (~88 per cent) or novice oarsmen (~65 per cent).

In the future, these types of measurements are likely to become popular for measuring the abilities of competitive rowers, especially if the information is made available in real-time for the rower. For example, by using a large visual display screen, information concerning unhelpful movement differences between the seat and handle during the early drive phase could be presented while rowing. Then any wasted slide length or early back extension errors could be measured and the information relayed to the display screen allowing alterations to be made on the next stroke. In this way, instrumented rowing machines could provide on-water rowers and coaches with a flexible training tool to enhance indoor rowing technique and improve on-water rowing technique.

At present, instrumented rowing machines are not widely available and those that do exist have usually been built for research purposes in universities or as personal engineering projects. For many years, the Austrian rowing company, WebaSport, did offer a product which allowed direct measurement of handle force and position for Concept2 machines. This useful system sold at a cost of around 1200 Euros and came with software which simplified data analysis. Unfortunately, it was discontinued in 2009. A Slovenian company, WiseCoach, has recently introduced their 4ROW system for use with a Concept2 machine. Strain gauges in the foot stretcher and handle as well as position sensors for the handle and seat provide a comprehensive set of measurements for analysing indoor rowing performance. Sadly, the high cost of this system is likely to exceed the budgets of most rowing programmes.

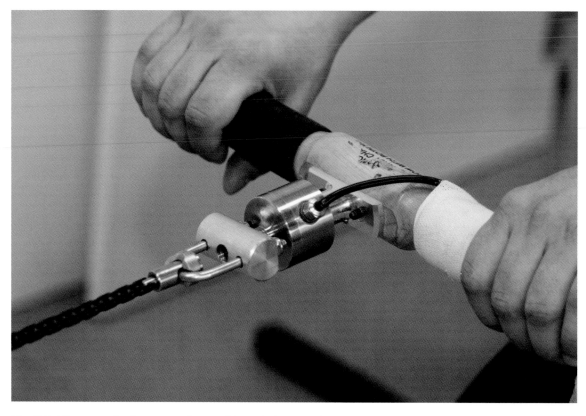

Fig 8.2 The use of a force transducer with an indoor rowing machine can provide additional information about a rower's technique

PEAK HANDLE FORCES AND DRAG FACTOR

There are consistent differences between force application patterns during the drive phase when using a stationary or sliding ergometer at the same overall power output. For example, force is developed quicker during the early part of the drive phase when rowing on a sliding ergometer. However, peak drive forces are between 5 and 10 per cent higher when using a stationary ergometer. The shape of the force curve during the drive phase is still reasonably similar between rowing on a stationary or sliding ergometer.

Considering that sliding ergometers were developed as a way to improve the dynamic feel of on-water rowing, it would be interesting to compare the handle forces of rowers during indoor and on-water rowing. Research provided by Dr Valery Kleshnev (www.biorow.com) has shown that peak handle forces are substantially higher during both stationary and sliding ergometer rowing in comparison with on-water sweep oar rowing (see figure 8.3). This difference is largely due to the effect of oar gearing. He also advises that rowers could improve the similarity between on-water and ergometer rowing by using low resistance settings (between position 1 and 5 on Models C, D and E) to reduce the drag factor (between 80 and 130). When attempting to simulate the dynamics of a coxed eight, the lowest lever position on a stationary ergometer should be used (1 to 2), whereas slower boats (e.g. single scull) can be better represented by a higher lever position (3 to 5). If a sliding or dynamic rowing ergometer is used in preference to a stationary ergometer, the resistance lever should be increased by an extra half unit to compensate for the slightly lower peak drive force that is typically observed during slide ergometer rowing (e.g. 4.5 versus 4.0).

The use of lower resistance settings may also reduce the risk of injury. Rowing machine use is often cited as a possible cause of back and rib injuries in on-water rowers and the drag forces

that are typically recommended may be too high. For example, the Concept2 Indoor Rowing Manual (Version 2) suggests that drag factors of 125 to 140 are typically suitable for training and testing of rowers aged 16 or older. However, many researchers now think that the use of lower drag factors during repetitive and prolonged ergometer rowing may help reduce the risk of injury by lowering the amount of strain placed on the musculoskeletal system. Indeed, Rowing Australia now encourage rowers to use sliding ergometers and to select lower drag factor settings to reduce injury risk (see figure 8.4). Their revised drag factor targets are clearly lower than previous recommendations and should result in handle forces and handle speeds that provide a better simulation of on-water rowing.

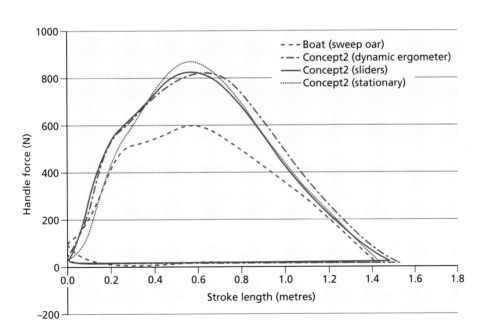

Fig 8.3 Comparison of handle force for on-water sweep oar rowing and for different indoor rowing machines (data courtesy of Dr Valery Kleshnev)

Category	Drag factor
Junior women	95
Lightweight women	95
Heavyweight women	105
Junior men	105
Lightweight men	105
Heavyweight men	115

Fig 8.4 Rowing Australia's recommended drag factor settings for 2000m competitive efforts when using a Concept2 indoor rowing machine with sliders

One concern that often prevents coaches and rowers from using lower drag factors of 80 to 120 units is that the physiological benefits of training may be compromised. However, researchers at Northern Michigan University reported that the acute physiological responses (oxygen consumption, heart rate and blood lactate) to rowing on a Concept2 ergometer were similar at drag factors of 100 and 150 units for 14 male and female college rowers. These provisional results suggest that low drag training may be suitable for promoting cardiovascular adaptations that are similar to those generated by higher drag settings. As mentioned earlier, the cardiovascular demands of stationary and slide ergometer rowing are also very similar. Thus, by lowering the injury risk and improving the similarity of indoor rowing to actual rowing, training outcomes for on-water rowers could be improved by emphasising the use of sliding ergometers with low drag factors in preference to stationary ergometer use with higher drag factors.

ARE 2000M PERFORMANCE TIMES ON STATIONARY AND SLIDING ROWING MACHINES DIFFERENT?

Given that there are several important mechanical differences between stationary and slide ergometer rowing, it would be interesting to know if 2000m performance times are also affected. There is some anecdotal evidence, especially from Australian rowing coaches, that the times of elite rowers are slightly faster when a sliding ergometer is used. However, the data presented by Kurt Jensen and colleagues in Denmark (described earlier) did not support a statistical difference in the 6 minute performance data of national team oarswomen when a stationary or sliding ergometer was used (295W versus 305W, respectively). To date, there has been no definitive answer offered by Concept2. Based on the available evidence, it seems likely that, on average, performance times will be similar on sliding and stationary machines. Possibly, elite rowers may gain a slight performance advantage from the use of sliding ergometers, whereas less skilful novice rowers may do better on a stationary machine. In both cases, the typical difference in time is likely to be very small and probably amounts to less than 1 per cent of 2000m time. For the time being, it is probably best to standardise all indoor rowing testing within a single season to one machine type regardless of whether a sliding or stationary ergometer is preferred.

DO INDOOR ROWING MACHINES PROVIDE A GOOD REPRESENTATION OF THE SKILL DEMANDS OF ON-WATER ROWING?

On-water rowers are often quick to suggest that skill is not an important consideration when using indoor rowing machines. Yet, non-rowers often struggle when they first begin indoor rowing training on any of the machines popularly used by on-water rowers. Effective rowing machine use does require the development of effective technique and it can take 2–3 months of regular training before a beginner reaches an acceptable skill level. Occasionally, a well-trained endurance athlete (e.g. swimmer, cyclist or runner), with less than 12 months of specific indoor rowing experience, is able to achieve a world class indoor rowing performance that is within 3 per cent of the 2000m Concept2 world record time in an open category. Normally, it takes between five and ten years of intense training to achieve a similar level of performance at a World Rowing Championship (on-water), although there are cases of exceptional athletes winning a senior world championship title after only two years of on-water training.

At a surface level, there is similarity between indoor and on-water rowing in terms of the lower body movements during the drive phase. Both types of rowing also require good suspension of body weight on the handle and excellent coordination between body segments. As a result, the patterns of force applied to the oar handles and ergometer handle appear reasonably similar. At the same time, there are important differences between machine and boat which should not be overlooked.

NEUROMUSCULAR SKILLS

Despite the apparent similarity in movement patterns between indoor and on-water rowing, the neuromuscular skills needed to reach an elite standard of on-water rowing are not fully challenged during ergometer rowing. Much of the apparent similarity in handle curves between ergometer and on-water rowing is misleading since these curves are created by distinct and different sequences of muscle fibre activations. In particular, the lack of any requirement to rotate the upper body during straight pull ergometer rowing substantially alters the neuromuscular similarities between on-water and indoor rowing. For sweep rowers in particular, these differences extend to the lower body since years of on-water rowing training result in different force contributions from the left and right leg, depending on which side the athlete rows. Ultimately, the ability of an indoor rowing machine to replicate the neuromuscular skills of on-water rowing is determined by how well the machine can replicate the actual oar trajectories. Additionally, the machine design must be able to replicate the typical handle speeds and resistance to movement encountered during on-water rowing in order to provide a closer approximation of the neuromuscular skills required in actual rowing. Clearly, there is much opportunity for future designers of rowing machines to better challenge the neuromuscular skills needed for successful on-water rowing.

BALANCE

Indoor rowing machines also struggle to simulate the technical demands of actual boat and oar handling. For example, modern rowing boats are unstable and mastering the skill of balancing a single scull takes many years of practice. Indoor rowing machines offer very limited challenge in terms of the balance skills need for on-water rowing. It is possible to purchase accessories such as the Core Perform seat (www.coreperform.com) which adds a small amount of balance challenge during indoor rowing. However, the demands of balancing a moving racing boat are complex and involve various interactions from the athlete, oars, environmental conditions and boat dynamics. These are extremely difficult to simulate on land and adding a seat-wobbling capability does very little to address the factors that influence boat balance. On-water rowing also requires a considerable amount of skill in oar handling which would also be extremely difficult to simulate on land.

Given the complex range of both neuromuscular and technical skill requirements involved in on-water rowing, building a rowing machine that provides a true simulation of on-water rowing is no easy feat. The current range of commercial rowing machines have far to go before they could truly be considered realistic simulators of the skill based demands of on-water rowing.

FUTURE DEVELOPMENTS IN ROWING SKILL SIMULATORS

Major improvements in the ability to simulate the demands of on-water rowing are certainly possible. In fact, it is conceivable that in the near future, rowing machines will develop into sophisticated simulators of on-water rowing that really do challenge the technical and neuromuscular skill of the user. These developments will first require computer software that is capable of modelling the various dynamic, kinematic and environmental interactions involved in on-water rowing. Hardware that incorporates rapid response sensors would then detect the actions of the indoor rower and simulate the responses that would occur during actual rowing. For example, changing the handle height during the drive phase would alter the amount of tilt applied to the simulator while pulling harder on the oar handle would increase the resistance to movement in a similar way to on-water efforts. Attempts to develop exactly these sorts of land-based rowing simulators using computer technology are currently well under way. Several research laboratories have made excellent advances in this area with computers already being used to stimulate the muscles of paraplegic individuals, making full body indoor rowing a possibility for wheelchair-bound individuals. While an indoor rowing machine that can truly replicate the experience and demands of on-water rowing may seem like science fiction, these types of advanced simulators are already proving their worth in Formula One motor racing. Potentially, the same technology that currently simulates the helmet forces experienced by racing drivers during a grand prix racing circuit may help develop indoor rowing machines that give a highly realistic representation of on-water rowing.

DO INDOOR ROWING MACHINES PROVIDE A GOOD REPRESENTATION OF THE PHYSIOLOGICAL DEMANDS OF ON-WATER ROWING?

National and international standard on-water rowers commonly spend between 20 and 40 per cent of their annual training time exercising on indoor rowing machines. Since these machines make relatively modest demands on the skill levels of rowers, it may be that the high investment of training time is better justified in terms of the related physiological adaptations. This issue has been the subject of many scientific investigations and good evidence shows broad agreement between various physiological responses that occur during a session of on-water rowing and responses to indoor rowing on Concept2, Gjessing and Rowperfect machines. It is important to note that these direct comparisons typically only consider the acute cardiovascular and blood lactate responses rather than the chronic changes following a period of prolonged training.

Scientists at the Australian Institute of Sport compared the physiological responses of seven national level male scullers during indoor rowing and on-water single sculling at matched power outputs. The athletes completed a series of 4 minute bouts of increasing intensity using a single scull or stationary Concept2 rowing machine until further bouts could not be performed due to fatigue. Power output during on-water sculling was measured using force transducers mounted in the sculling oarlocks. Sub-maximal physiological responses, including average heart rate, blood lactate and oxygen consumption, were similar between on-water and indoor rowing when compared at similar power output values. During the final 4 minute bout (maximal effort) only heart rate was statistically different with slightly lower values record during sculling (188 beats per minute) versus ergometer rowing (192 beats per minute). There were no differences in maximum lactate or maximum oxygen consumption. These results show that the patterns of physiological responses are broadly similar during on-water sculling and indoor rowing, at least when standard physiological measurements are used. The researchers also noticed that although the average responses of the group were similar, some individual athletes displayed considerable variation between their physiological measurements obtained during on-water and ergometer rowing. This study is particularly helpful since the comparisons were made at similar power outputs and not matched velocities or stroke rates, which is the usual approach of researchers. When the distances completed in each 4 minute bout were compared, the Concept2 performance monitor significantly overestimated the actual distance of sculling (calm water conditions). During the maximal effort stage, average distances completed were 1040m for single sculling and 1267m for stationary rowing on the Concept2 ergometer.

MUSCLE FIBRE RESPONSES

While standard physiological measurements are relatively similar between indoor rowing and on-water rowing, there are a number of other important physiological measures that have not been investigated. In particular, the extent to which indoor and on-water rowing stimulates similar physiological responses at the level of individual muscle fibres has not been well studied.

Based on the differences in movement patterns noted earlier for land-based and water-based rowing, it is highly likely that substantial differences in specific muscle fibre adaptations occur. It is at least possible to speculate that the magnitude of the difference should be reduced if a circular pull rowing machine is used instead of a straight pull machine, however, the effects of these changes on 2000m on-water performance are not known.

USAGE PATTERNS OF INDOOR ROWING MACHINES DURING A COMPETITIVE ROWING SEASON

The usual pattern of indoor rowing machine use during a competitive training programme involves high amounts of ergometer training in the early and middle parts of the season (preparation phase), before machine use is substantially reduced or eliminated during the competitive on-water phase. The pattern of ergometer use will also be influenced by the prevailing weather conditions during each part of the training year. In the northern hemisphere, ergometer training volumes are highest between October and March, and it is during this period that athletes are most likely to achieve personal best ergometer performances. Thereafter, on-water training typically takes priority and as a consequence of the reduced amount of training time spent on rowing machines, ergometer time trial performances tend to plateau and on-water monitoring of performance becomes more important.

At the international level, it is not uncommon for on-water rowers to continue with regular ergometer training right up until the final weeks before the World Championships. This may help preserve baseline aerobic fitness, add variety to training and possibly improve the ability to detect early signs of overtraining. On the other hand, rowers competing at national standard or below are likely to have lower technical proficiency and overall training volumes. These rowers will probably gain better on-water results from directing their limited available training time during the racing season to boat-specific conditioning, possibly to the total exclusion of any ergometer training or testing.

DOES INDOOR ROWING PERFORMANCE PREDICT ON-WATER ROWING PERFORMANCE?

The introduction of the Concept2 Model B rowing machine, complete with programmable LCD screen, triggered a major shift in crew selection procedures. Coaches and team selectors were able to justify their crew selections, in part, based on an athlete's 2500m or 2000m ergometer test result. Of course, many on-water rowers were unimpressed and frequently objected to selection by erg score or simply objected to a selector's use of the results. The extract below is taken from an open letter that was published in a popular rowing magazine in 2001. The letter was directed to the selectors of the United States national rowing team and makes clear several common frustrations and objections to ergometer testing:

'We need to replace the present emphasis on raw ergometer scores with weight-adjusted scores. The problems with ergometer scores are well known:

they reward excess weight and ignore technique. Because scores are the basis for nearly every invitation to [selection] camps, potentially excellent competitors are being passed by. Every coach has discovered that a boat of top erg scores is frequently beaten by the next set of scorers, and they eventually compose their top boat by seat racing and technique observations. But you cannot seat-race people who aren't there.'

(Source: *Independent Rowing News*, October 2001)

The use of rowing machines for athlete selection remains a contentious issue but usually only at the club and university level (sub-elite). International rowers generally appreciate and accept the need for ergometer selection tests and most national team selection procedures require that rowers complete an ergometer time trial at different stages in the process. For example, any rower seeking selection for the British rowing team must first perform a mandatory and publically witnessed 2000m ergometer trial. Only rowers who achieve the published minimum ergometer times are allowed to compete in the subsequent on-water tests. No weight-adjusted procedures are used, but lightweight competitors have a separate minimum score according to their category (e.g. under 23 or open). Interestingly, national team selectors and top coaches often take special interest in any trialist who demonstrates exceptional indoor rowing performance but fails to achieve a high standard of on-water performance. These rowers are likely to be given encouragement to relocate to a high performance training centre or offered alternative fast track activities to improve their on-water ability.

At the elite level, indoor rowing performance is clearly valued as one important indicator of on-water performance potential. Many national rowing federations now include specific 2000m Concept2 ergometer times in their international selection documents. Closer examination of these times reveals slight differences in the approaches taken by each federation. For example, Rowing Australia lists benchmark times for senior athletes that they believe will be necessary for athletes to medal at the Olympics. On the other hand, British Rowing prefer to list the minimum qualifying standard required for entry to the formal selection process. Figure 8.5 provides a list of the benchmark or minimum qualifying standards for a selection of international rowing teams based on their official selection policy documents (2010–2011 season).

Why then does the inclusion of ergometer test data still cause considerable controversy over athlete selection at the sub-elite level? One likely explanation is that there is simply less understanding and awareness of the value and limitations of ergometer data at this level. As described earlier, indoor rowing machines are relatively poor simulators of the skill demands of on-water racing, but are reasonably good at simulating the physiological demands. While it is difficult to estimate the exact contributions of a rower's skill or physiological abilities to their 2000m on-water performance, it is possible that many coaches and rowers overestimate the importance of skill and underestimate the importance of physiology. After all, it is much easier to observe the technique of a rower than it is their heart size, blood volume or other important physiological feature. Also, rowing coaches frequently spend huge amounts of time stressing the need for their rowers to pay close

		Benchmark standards			Minimum qualifying standards	
		Australia*	New Zealand	United States	Ireland	Great Britain
Men	Heavyweight	5:48	5:54	6:00	6:10	6:10
	Lightweight	6:08	6:13	6:14	6:36	6:33
	Heavyweight (U-23)	5:53	6:01	6:04	6:19	6:20
	Lightweight (U-23)	6:14	6:17	6:18	6:45	6:43
	Junior	6:11	6:12	6:20	6:55	6:55
		Australia*	New Zealand	United States	Ireland	Great Britain
Women	Heavyweight	6:40	6:49	6:45	7:00	7:05
	Lightweight	7:00	7:10	7:10	7:38	7:28
	Heavyweight (U-23)	6:46	6:57	6:55	7:10	7:15
	Lightweight (U-23)	7:06	7:17	7:15	7:49	7:38
	Junior	7:06	7:12	7:15	7:50	7:20

*Rowing Australia now require athletes to test on Concept2 sliders

Fig 8.5 Comparison of the 2000m Concept2 ergometer times of various international rowing teams. Benchmark standards are times that are likely to be required to either gain selection to the national team or to medal at Olympic level. Minimum qualifying standards are required in order to proceed to advanced stages of selection.

attention to the details of their stroke technique. It's quite possible that these issues may be responsible for a certain amount of inflation in the minds of many coaches and rowers at the sub-elite level about the importance of technique for determining on-water performance.

In contrast, national team selectors and elite coaches typically have a more sophisticated understanding of the factors that limit on-water performance, in part, because of better access to sport science support as well as extensive experience of working with top athletes who are reasonably similar in terms of fitness and skill levels.

'ERGS DON'T FLOAT'

Another reason why some coaches and rowers may downplay the predictive value of ergometer test scores may be explained by the popular phrase, 'ergs don't float'. This phrase is often used in reference to an individual who displays exceptional indoor rowing performance, but generally fails to score well during on-water assessments. The powerful imagery of this phrase is often supported with stories about exceptional indoor rowers who were unsuccessful in on-water competitions such as the German rower Matthias Siejkowski. Matthias established himself as a legend of indoor rowing, winning numerous indoor titles and setting multiple world records in the 1990s, including a 5:37 in the open men's 2000m event. Many observers assumed that the combination of his incredible ergometer ability and 208cm height would surely translate into major success in on-water competitions. Matthias did race in several international regattas, including the World

Championships, but with largely unremarkable results. Proponents of the 'ergs don't float' argument can usually provide similar stories of local or international rowers who struggled to keep their on-water rowing career afloat despite maintaining a perfectly buoyant indoor rowing ability.

There are many world class indoor rowers who have never set foot in a competitive racing boat. These individuals would undoubtedly do very poorly, at least at first, if imported directly into a competitive crew. But this is not a good argument to abandon the use of indoor rowing trials as part of crew selection procedures. Since on-water rowers are often most interested in world class on-water rowing performance, it is better to examine the ergometer scores of the best on-water rowers to see if these athletes also have outstanding abilities on rowing machines. In fact, there is good general support for this position providing that any such comparison is made using national and international level rowers. Comparisons of indoor and on-water rowing performance, when made at relatively low levels of rowing ability, are less helpful due to the large number of potentially limiting factors. When developing a comprehensive selection policy, coaches who predominantly work with novice and intermediate level rowers should first assess the basic on-water skills of each rower before turning their attention toward the results of indoor rowing tests. When levels of rowing skill become more homogenous, such as in a group of well-trained on-water rowers, indoor rowing scores more clearly emerge as a useful way to predict differences in on-water performance.

Various researchers have compared the 2000m indoor and on-water rowing performances of national and international standard rowers. Some of these studies found that ergometer performance was a good predictor of on-water performance, while others found no clear relationship. These equivocal results are probably due to the limitations of using small groups of only 10–20 rowers to make the statistical comparisons, as well as using a diverse range of rowing ability. When there are only a small number of observations to compare, there is a much greater chance that one or two extreme performances will have a disproportionate effect. A good way to understand the relationship between ergometer scores and on-water performances is to examine these relationships in a large sample of highly trained on-water rowers.

Researchers from Croatia were able to obtain information about the ergometer scores of the majority of competitors at both the 2007 World Junior and World Senior Rowing Championships. Athletes at these events completed a survey of their personal rowing background, body size and best 2000m performance on a Concept2 stationary ergometer in 2007. The researchers then compared the information provided by the rowers to their final on-water rank order according to their specific boat class. The average 2000m ergometer times are provided in figure 8.6 according to the classification of athlete.

The analysis and interpretation of the data for the larger boat classes is complicated due to missing data and a smaller range of possible crew rankings, but a clear and consistent picture does emerge from examination of small boat data, especially the single sculls. Across all the different single scull divisions at world senior and junior rowing championships, self-reported 2000m ergometer scores explained approximately 60 per cent of the variation in on-water single scull performance. The highest relationship was

	Heavyweight		Lightweight		Junior	
	Men	Women	Men	Women	Men	Women
2000m time (minutes:seconds)	6:04	6:56	6:23	7:17	6:27	7:25
Number of rowers in sample	230	137	156	137	222	160

Fig 8.6 Self-reported 2000m ergometer times of competitors at the FISA 2007 Senior and Junior World Rowing Regatta (adapted from Mikulic et al., 2009)

observed for the junior women single scullers, where ergometer scores explained 85 per cent of the variation in final championship placing. Conversely, the lowest relationship was observed for the lightweight women's single scullers, where ergometer scores explained 45 per cent of the variation in final championship rank order.

Although the results of these large-scale analyses from regattas provide a clearer understanding of the extent to which 2000m indoor rowing scores can accurately predict the on-water performance of skilled rowers, they are not definitive. Importantly, the use of simple correlation-based analysis can be misleading since other variables may confound the interpretation. For example, training volume and employment status may partly explain some of the observed relationship between ergometer and on-water performance since top international rowers are likely to perform very high volumes of both on-water and indoor rowing as part of their annual training time. The highest training volumes are likely to be performed by full time rowers who receive funding to train. These individuals are then able to perform more on-water and indoor training, resulting in better performances in both types of rowing. Future studies may help refine the predictive value of indoor rowing testing, but on the basis of the

available evidence, the practice of including ergometer trial data as part of crew selection procedures is well supported.

RELIABILITY OF PERFORMANCE TESTS USING ROWING MACHINES

Trained rowers are capable of repeating 2000m time trial performances with extremely high levels of consistency from day to day. Researchers in South Africa compared 2000m indoor rowing performance of eight well-trained schoolboy rowers on three occasions with at least 3 days between tests. All testing was conducted at the same time of day and both the training and diet of the rowers were controlled in the days before each test. After a 5 minute warm-up on a Concept2 ergometer, the rowers completed a 2000m time trial but were only able to see the distance remaining and stroke rate on the performance monitor. The performances were highly correlated and average times were 6:56, 6:54 and 6:51 for the first, second and third days, respectively. The slight improvement over the 3 days suggests that the rowers were gaining confidence in their pacing ability at each successive test. It is likely that time trial performances would be even more similar if the additional pacing feedback from the performance monitor was provided.

Separate research at the Australian Institute of Sport with national level rowers also showed that time trial performance and physiological responses are highly reproducible on different days, even when using different Concept2 models (Model C versus Model D), providing that the drag factor was standardised. Overall, the 2000m indoor rowing performance times of trained rowers typically vary by as little as 0.5–1.0 per cent between days and show remarkable stability. This high reliability of indoor rowing performance testing makes it much easier for coaches and athletes to assess the effects of acute interventions such as trialing a new type of nutrition supplement or training device.

GUIDANCE FOR SETTING ERGOMETER TIME STANDARDS

Despite the available evidence that ergometer performances provide a reliable and valid indication of a rower's on-water performance, it may be easiest for coaches who work with large teams of rowers to set ergometer performance standards for crew selection. Since success in major on-water rowing events at national and international level is related to the average ergometer score of a crew, much of the controversy inherent in crew selection can be reduced if the coach stipulates a minimum ergometer score necessary for selection in advance.

Each coach will need to select their minimum score with care, and where possible, obtain trustworthy information about the average ergometer scores of recent winners in the target event. For example, international success in a men's heavyweight eight is likely to require a crew where all rowers can achieve a 2000m time of 6:05, whereas success at Henley Royal Regatta in the men's club eights (Thames Challenge Cup) or student eights (Temple Challenge Cup) is likely to require all rowers to achieve a 2000m time of 6:20. The use of minimum targets makes it easier for a coach to quickly reduce a large pool of rowers to a manageable number from which further assessments of boat moving ability (e.g. seat-racing) should be used. Irrespective of the performance level selected, it is important to publicise these targets to all rowers early in the season. This encourages rowers to take their ergometer training seriously and provides a smoother path for coaches at the first selection point. While absolute cut-offs are easy for all rowers to understand, their usefulness in predicting on-water performances is greatest when all members of a crew have reasonably similar body weights. If sizeable differences in body weights do exist, then the use of weight-adjusted ergometer scores are likely to give better estimates of on-water potential and may be worth considering.

WEIGHT-ADJUSTED ERGOMETER SCORES

The difference in 2000m race performance between top lightweight and heavyweight competitors is approximately 7.5 per cent for indoor rowing compared to only 2.5 per cent for on-water racing. The smaller performance gap during on-water rowing is mostly due to the extra drag created by the need for the boats of heavyweight rowers to displace more water than the boats of lightweight rowers. In fact, the gap in on-water performance could probably be reduced further if minimum boat and cox weights were set as a proportion of crew weight rather than a fixed minimum. Under such circumstances, heavyweight rowers would still retain a small advantage due to their greater anaerobic power which is proportional to absolute muscle mass. In any event, adjusting 2000m ergometer scores to control for the added drag penalty due to increases in body weight is a straightforward procedure.

Since body weight is still an important determinant of on-water performance, adjusting ergometer performance scores to completely remove size differences would be unhelpful. Instead, the relationship between ergometer speed and boat speed can be mathematically modelled and the results used to create a formula which corrects for the effect of body weight. For example, Concept2 offer an online weight adjustment calculator (http://www.concept2.com/us/interactive/calculators/) which transforms a 2000m ergometer score into an equivalent 2000m on-water time for a coxed eight assuming all rowers have the same body weight and ergometer time. The predicted on-water times for a range of ergometer performances and body weights are shown in figure 8.7.

Using the expected crew average for 2000m ergometer scores of top lightweight and heavyweight oarsmen, we can compare the predicted results of an on-water race using the Concept2 formula. If we assume that a top lightweight crew is likely to have a 2000m average ergometer performance of 6:15 and a crew weight of 70kg, whereas a top heavyweight crew is likely to average 6:00 and weigh at least 85kg, the predicted on-water times of these racing eights, assuming ideal conditions and excellent technique, are 5:31 for the lightweights and 5:32 for the heavyweights. These simulated results are reasonably similar to the actual performances of top lightweight and heavyweight eights at world rowing championships. This procedure should work equally well with female or junior rowers.

Calculating weight-adjusted 2000m times

Use the calculator found at http://www.concept2.com/us/interactive/calculators/

Step 1: Calculate weight correction factor as [body weight in kg / 122.5kg] raised to the power 0.222

Step 2: Multiply weight-corrected factor by unadjusted score on Concept2 for 2000m

(Note: If using Imperial units, then change Step 1 as follows: Calculate weight correction factor as [body weight in lbs / 270lbs] raised to the power 0.222)

Weight kg (lbs)	2000m score on stationary Concept2 rowing machine (unadjusted)													Predicted on-water time in a sweep Eight over 2000m*
	5:30	5:45	6:00	6:15	6:30	6:45	7:00	7:15	7:30	7:45	8:00	8:15	8:30	
55 (121)	4:36	4:49	5:01	5:14	5:26	5:39	5:51	6:04	6:17	6:29	6:42	6:54	7:07	
60 (132)	4:42	4:54	5:07	5:20	5:33	5:46	5:58	6:11	6:24	6:37	6:49	7:02	7:15	
65 (143)	4:47	5:00	5:13	5:26	5:39	5:52	6:05	6:18	6:31	6:44	6:57	7:10	7:23	
70 (154)	4:51	5:05	5:18	5:31	5:44	5:58	6:11	6:24	6:37	6:51	7:04	7:17	7:30	
75 (165)	4:56	5:09	5:23	5:36	5:50	6:03	6:17	6:30	6:43	6:57	7:10	7:24	7:37	
80 (176)	5:00	5:14	5:27	5:41	5:55	6:08	6:22	6:36	6:49	7:03	7:16	7:30	7:44	
85 (187)	5:04	5:18	5:32	5:46	5:59	6:13	6:27	6:41	6:55	7:09	7:22	7:36	7:50	
90 (198)	5:08	5:22	5:36	5:50	6:04	6:18	6:32	6:46	7:00	7:14	7:28	7:42	7:56	
95 (209)	5:12	5:26	5:40	5:54	6:08	6:23	6:37	6:51	7:05	7:19	7:33	7:48	8:02	
100 (220)	5:15	5:30	5:44	5:58	6:13	6:27	6:41	6:56	7:10	7:24	7:39	7:53	8:07	

*Assumes ideal environmental conditions and excellent technique

Fig 8.7 Weight-adjusted 2000m times on a Concept2 indoor rowing machine for a range of different body weights

Summary

In closing, it is clear that ergometer scores can help coaches to make initial judgements about the on-water potential of a rower. Nevertheless, coaches still need to be careful to avoid over-reliance on the quantitative data available from rowing machines. On-water rowing performance is also influenced by how well matched a crew is and how well they handle different water conditions. The subjective opinion of an experienced coach is still likely to provide the best solution to the problems of crew selection. On-water seat racing is still useful, but coaches should be mindful that the day-to-day variability in on-water crew performance is typically greater than for ergometer tests and this makes it harder to detect clear differences between individuals.

Rowing machines have become essential to both the training and testing of on-water rowers across all ability levels, and may become even more important in future years with further advances in technology and machine design.

NUTRITION FOR INDOOR ROWING

9

Nutrition plays an important role in determining a person's health and physical performance. However, making even relatively minor changes to a person's usual diet can be a substantial challenge. Most indoor rowers will already be familiar with much of the standard nutrition advice that is supplied by government health agencies and major nutrition organisations. The information provided in national health campaigns to reduce soft drink consumption or lower daily salt intake is just as important to indoor rowers as it is to untrained individuals. Regular exercise can deliver some of the same benefits from eating a healthy diet (e.g. improved body weight control), but in many cases the positive health effects from good nutrition are added to the positive effects of regular physical activity. Equally, there are limits to the benefits of exercise. In many instances, the significant damage caused by years of poor dietary choices cannot simply be undone by regular physical activity, no matter how hard or how long a person exercises. It is not the purpose of this book to review and repackage this broad nutrition advice. Instead, we simply wish to make clear that it would be a serious mistake to believe that regular exercise is sufficient to compensate for poor dietary choices.

This chapter focuses on specific nutrition information and advice that is of direct relevance to indoor rowers, particularly indoor rowers who are training for competition. We begin by discussing nine important suggestions concerning different ways that indoor rowers can use nutrition to support the demands of regular training. Next, we briefly consider some of the unique problems faced by lightweight competitors when attempting weight loss. In the final section of this chapter, we explore the fascinating subject of using nutritional supplements to improve to 2000m indoor rowing performance.

NUTRITION SUGGESTIONS FOR INDOOR ROWING TRAINING
TRAINING SUGGESTION #1: ENSURE AN APPROPRIATE DAILY CALORIC INTAKE TO ACHIEVE TRAINING AND WEIGHT LOSS GOALS

The best estimates of the daily energy intake requirements of adults suggest that the typical women needs to consume 2000kcal per day, while the typical man needs to consume 2500kcal per day. These levels are considered suitable to maintain stable body weight and good health. However, these values assume normal body size and relatively low daily activity levels. Since indoor rowers often have higher daily activity levels than the typical adult, higher energy intakes are usually required, especially for indoor rowers with body weights above typical values (i.e. women >65kg and men >85kg).

For recreational indoor rowers who achieve the recommended weekly amounts of physical activity (i.e. 150 minutes of moderate intensity exercise), the modest increase in daily energy requirement is usually balanced by a slight increase in appetite. Providing that body weight is stable and at the desired level, there is usually no need for recreational rowers to make conscious effort to alter daily energy intake levels. However, competitive indoor rowers completing between 30 and 100km (or more) of weekly indoor rowing are likely to require increases in daily energy intake by as much as 10 to 100 per cent above typical values.

The appetite of competitive indoor rowers will usually change to suit alterations to their daily energy intake requirements. However, there are circumstances where appetite will be a poor guide for determining daily energy needs and specific conscious effort is needed to achieve training and body composition goals. For example, indoor rowers who perform very high volumes of training may underestimate their energy needs due to the appetite suppressing effects of exercise and the desire to avoid training on a heavy stomach. Also, appetite will be a poor guide for the indoor rower who is attempting to reduce body weight by increasing the amount of training and reducing energy intake. Unless a sustained conscious effort is made to override the increase in hunger from a persistent energy deficit, the rower will be unable to achieve their weight loss goals due to excessive food intake. These are complex issues due to the wide range of individual training circumstances and difficulties in controlling eating behaviour.

> Indoor rowers with heavy training loads and/ or attempting significant weight loss should consult a qualified sport nutritionist to obtain an accurate estimate of their daily energy needs and to develop a personalised eating plan that can meet their individual training and lifestyle preferences.

For most competitive indoor rowers, the rowing machine monitor will provide a reasonable estimate of the extra energy expenditure from each training session. These values provide a useful starting point for calculating additional energy needs above typical daily amounts. One simple way to estimate the appropriateness of an indoor rower's daily energy balance is to check if body weight remains stable over time. When measured under controlled conditions, body weight fluctuates by less than 1kg per day. If body weight is increasing or decreasing by more than this amount, then too much or too little energy is being consumed, respectively, for the level of training and should be adjusted. In circumstances where relatively minor reductions in body weight loss are desired (i.e. 1–5kg reductions), conscious efforts to reduce the fat content of an indoor rower's diet can help produce a suitable energy deficit without significantly compromising training capacity.

TRAINING SUGGESTION #2: CONSUME A LEVEL OF DAILY CARBOHYDRATE INTAKE THAT IS SUITABLE FOR YOUR LEVEL OF TRAINING

There is good evidence to suggest that competitive indoor rowers can benefit from increasing daily carbohydrate intake. Carbohydrate is the most important fuel source during moderate and high intensity rowing, but the amounts stored in the human body are relatively small. Carbohydrate reserves can be depleted after just 90 minutes of moderate intensity indoor rowing, or after just 20 minutes of high intensity interval training. An inadequate daily intake of carbohydrate can reduce endurance capacity and significantly restrict the ability to perform moderate and high intensity rowing.

Indoor rowers need to make sure to consume enough carbohydrate to avoid the problems of carbohydrate depletion, but this can be a considerable challenge. It is usually impractical to complete a full dietary profile to determine the per cent of carbohydrate in an indoor rower's diet. Instead, a more user-friendly solution is to select a relative amount of carbohydrate intake (g per kg body weight) which is appropriate to training level. Figure 9.1 provides a list of daily carbohydrate intake targets that are suitable for different levels of training. For example, a 60kg female who rows

60km per week should aim to consume between 300 and 420g of carbohydrate per day (i.e. 5–7g of carbohydrate per kg body weight).

Research studies that provide a direct comparison of the effects of daily carbohydrate intake levels on exercise training and performance gains are extremely rare. However, one of the only studies to consider this issue was performed by researchers at Ohio State University who examined the effects of two different levels of daily carbohydrate intake on the ability of rowers to complete a 28 day period of indoor rowing training.

Male and female university rowers (N=22) volunteered to complete an extremely difficult training program that consisted of two indoor rowing sessions every day for 6 days per week. Rowers were randomly assigned to either a moderate carbohydrate group (5g per kg body weight per day; 42 per cent of daily energy intake) or a high carbohydrate group (10g per kg body weight per day; 70 per cent of daily energy intake). The researchers provided all the necessary dietary requirements to meet the individual needs of each rower. Additionally, rowers in the high carbohydrate group received liquid meal supplements to boost total carbohydrate intake, whereas the moderate carbohydrate group consumed additional fat to ensure that the total energy intake of both groups was identical.

Standard of training	Weekly volume of rowing (km)	Recommended daily carbohydrate target (grams of carbohydrate per kg of body weight)
Basic	<40	3 to 5
Intermediate	40 to 80	5 to 7
Advanced	>80	7 to 12

Fig 9.1 Daily carbohydrate intake targets for indoor rowers based on weekly training volume

All rowers completed the same training programme using a Concept2 machine. Sessions were performed at either moderate or high intensities and included an interval session of 3 x 2500m maximal effort intervals with 8 minute rest periods every Monday, Wednesday and Friday. At the end of the four week programme, average power output during the final 2500m interval session had improved by 2 per cent in the moderate carbohydrate group compared to 11 per cent improvement in the high carbohydrate group. Using muscle tissue samples taken from the legs of the rowers, the researchers demonstrated that the high carbohydrate group were able to store more glucose in their leg muscles than the moderate carbohydrate group. They suggested that the differences in carbohydrate availability during training explained the improved training and final performance abilities of the high carbohydrate group.

These results provide good evidence to suggest that adjusting daily carbohydrate intake levels can improve indoor rowing training and performance, at least during prolonged periods of very intense and demanding training. However, very high levels of daily carbohydrate intake would be excessive to the needs of most indoor rowers and may even be detrimental to performance due to unwanted weight gain. Nutrition surveys of recreational, club and elite athletes suggest that men are typically better than women at meeting carbohydrate targets similar to those outlined in figure 9.1. At the same time, most indoor rowers will receive health benefits, and possibly some performance benefits, by making minor reductions in their daily fat intake along with proportional increases in daily carbohydrate intake to match the recommendations outlined above.

TRAINING SUGGESTION #3: MAINTAIN GOOD HYDRATION BEFORE, DURING AND AFTER TRAINING

Dehydration is well known to influence performance in athletic events that last several minutes or longer. Endurance capacity is noticeably compromised when fluid losses exceed approximately 2 per cent of body weight. For a 60kg individual, 2 per cent dehydration is equivalent to a 1.2kg decrease in body weight. Typically, when dehydration is present before exercise it is usually explained by insufficient food and drink consumption. Even when an indoor rower begins exercise well hydrated, significant dehydration can develop due to high rates of sweat loss. Typical sweat rates during moderate intensity indoor rowing are usually between 1 and 2 litres per hour. Higher absolute sweat rates are likely when rowing is performed in hot conditions, when higher exercise intensity is used and for individuals with large body size.

Based on the limited research that has been conducted with indoor rowing performance, we estimate that 2000m indoor rowing times will be approximately 0.5–3 per cent slower when an indoor rower begins a 2000m race with a level of dehydration between 2 and 5 per cent. Thus, an indoor rower who can achieve a 2000m time of exactly 7 minutes when normally hydrated would extend their race time by as much as 2–13 seconds if dehydration of between 2 and 5 per cent was present.

Calculating sweat loss and dehydration during rowing

Based on the knowledge that 1 litre of sweat weighs 1kg, indoor rowers can estimate total sweat loss during indoor rowing by comparing pre- and post-training body weight measurements. You will need to ensure that you make a like-for-like body weight assessment. One way to do this is to empty your bladder, take a quick shower, and then towel dry as best as possible before obtaining the pre-exercise weight measurement while nude or wearing dry clothing. There will still be small amounts of water on your skin and in your hair but don't worry about these. Complete your rowing training, taking note of any quantities of fluid that you consumed, then repeat the showering and weighing process. Make sure to dry yourself as well as before and then to take the body weight measurement nude or wearing the exact same dry clothing as before. If you wear your sweaty rowing outfit you will underestimate your fluid loss since some of your sweat loss will be trapped in your clothes.

Total sweat losses are calculated by subtracting post-training body weight from pre-training body weight. If you consumed any fluids between weight measurements, then you also need to remove the weight of this fluid from the post-weight value for the purposes of calculating your total sweat loss. For example, if your pre-training weight was 60kg and your post-training weight was 59kg and you ingested 500ml of fluid during training (i.e. 0.5kg), your adjusted post-exercise body weight is actually 58.5kg. The 1.5kg weight change is your total sweat loss and represents the total amount of fluid that you would need to drink during training to completely offset exercise-induced dehydration. If we assume that you started the session with normal hydration, then total sweat losses were enough to generate a 2.5 per cent level of dehydration by the end of exercise (1.5kg divided by 60kg x 100). You replaced 0.5kg of sweat loss by drinking during

training, so your actual level of dehydration after exercise was only 1.7 per cent (1.0 kg divided by 60 kg x 100). Therefore, you only replaced 33 per cent of your total sweat losses during training but had not quite reached the 2 per cent level of dehydration where performance is generally considered to be adversely affected.

Calculating sweat loss

Sweat loss during training (kg) = (Pre-training weight (kg) – post-training weight (kg)) + fluid ingested during training (kg)

Dehydration can reduce training and performance. Dehydration can also make training feel harder and increases the risk of heat stress. There is no clear benefit to overhydrating so a sensible approach to hydration is to ensure that you begin training appropriately hydrated and then to drink during training according to thirst levels, while ensuring sufficient fluid intake to limit exercise-induced dehydration to less than 2 per cent.

Maintaining proper hydration levels

Pre-exercise

- At least 4 hours before exercise:
  - slowly drink a moderate amount of fluid (5 to 7ml/kg of body weight).
- Approximately 2 hours before exercise:
  - check urine production – if no urine is produced or is darkly coloured then continue to slowly drink a smaller amount of fluid (3 to 5ml/kg of body weight) and

- continue to monitor fluid intake until the start of training, drinking small quantities of water or sports drinks according to personal preference.
- Avoid any attempt to overhydrate by consuming large quantities of fluid.
- Water or sports drinks are both appropriate pre-exercise fluid choices.

During exercise

- Develop an awareness of your typical sweat rates during indoor rowing by making suitable comparisons of pre- and post-exercise body weight in training.
- Try to limit exercise-induced dehydration to less than 2 per cent of normal body weight by taking regular drink breaks. If you do not want to stop rowing to drink, consider the use of a specialist fluid backpack with a drinking tube.
- Sports drinks or water are both suitable choices.

After exercise

- Normal fluid and food consumption is usually sufficient for rehydration.
- If more aggressive rehydration is required, consume 1.5 litres of fluid for each kilogram of body weight lost due to exercise and consider consuming salty snacks to stimulate thirst.
- Sports drinks or water are both suitable choices.

(Modified from: American College of Sports Medicine's Exercise and Fluid Replacement Position Stand, 2007)

TRAINING SUGGESTION #4: ENHANCE RECOVERY FROM TRAINING BY CONSUMING CARBOHYDRATE SOON AFTER EXERCISE

For competitive indoor rowers performing moderate and high training loads, it is important to restore carbohydrate losses as soon as reasonably possible to ensure that performance at the next training session is not compromised due to reduced energy stores. For most rowers, the best way to do this is to simply eat their next meal at the earliest opportunity. However, eating soon after training may not be convenient and appetite is often reduced for several hours due to changes in the release of hormones that control hunger levels. A good solution is to bring a carbohydrate-rich snack to a training session (e.g. fruit, vegetables, chocolate, sports bar or sports drinks). This may take a little more planning, but there are plenty of benefits to making a little extra effort before and after training.

If food intake is delayed for several hours after prolonged exercise the rate of muscle glycogen restoration will be slower than if food is eaten soon after exercise. The best way to ensure that muscle carbohydrate levels are quickly replaced after training is to consume 50g or more of carbohydrate within 30 minutes after exercise. The importance of more aggressive carbohydrate replacement strategies depends on the volume, intensity and frequency of your training. Fast rates of carbohydrate replacement are of greatest importance after high volume or high intensity training and when training will be repeated at intervals of 24 hours or less. Indoor rowers who regularly complete high training loads for several days at a time can improve overall training capacity by paying attention to both the total daily intake of carbohydrate (discussed earlier) as well as how quickly carbohydrate is consumed after training.

TRAINING SUGGESTION #5: REDUCE THE RISK OF ILLNESS DURING TRAINING THROUGH GOOD PRACTICE AND PROVIDING KEY NUTRIENTS KNOWN TO IMPROVE HEALTH

Indoor rowers can easily pick up bacteria and viruses from the machine handle. Use of a rowing machine in a boathouse or gym is likely to increase your risk of catching an illness due to the use of shared machines. The large number of rowers who continue to train with open blisters across their hands often makes the contamination problem even worse. It is also very easy to transfer bugs from the handle of the machine to the lid of a drink bottle, which then allows the bacteria or viruses to enter the body and spread infection. Sharing drink bottles is another way that indoor rowers unwittingly increase their risk of illness. By improving basic hygiene, such as cleaning the machine handle before and after training, indoor rowers can reduce the risk of infection. Avoid the practice of sharing drink bottles and be sure to wash drink bottles properly between uses.

Another good way to reduce illness risk is to ensure a good supply of several important nutrients. Carbohydrate intake during, and immediately after exercise, is a well-established way to boost immune function and reduce infection risk. Consuming a standard sports drink (6 per cent carbohydrate solution such as Lucozade, Powerade or Gatorade) reduces cortisol release and improves cytokine availability (cytokines are protein based molecules secreted by immune cells which trigger physiological changes in a similar way to hormones). There doesn't seem to be any additional benefit from consuming more highly-concentrated sports drinks or sports gels (e.g. 12 per cent carbohydrate). The selective use of certain vitamin and mineral supplements may also be helpful to immune function. For example, a major scientific review suggests that zinc ingestion, when taken within the first 24 hours after common cold symptoms begin, appears to slightly reduce the duration and severity of the illness. However, regular consumption does not reduce an adult's risk of developing the common cold.

One way that indoor rowers often try to reduce their illness risk is through the use of a multi-vitamin or multi-mineral supplement. This may provide short-term benefits to health and immune function during periods of high load training or when daily food is restricted, such as when attempting to reduce body weight. Typically, it is better to achieve the recommended intake levels of vitamins and minerals by consuming a diet that is high in fruits and vegetables. Habitual use of vitamin and mineral supplements increases the risk of over-consumption and this may actually reduce training adaptations by disrupting metabolic signals that are responsible for training adaptions. Researchers have only recently started to investigate this issue, but there are reasonable speculations that the normal inflammatory effects of exercise, which produce free radicals, are actually an important part of the conditioning process. Consuming anti-inflammatory nutrition supplements such as vitamin C and vitamin E can reduce free radical availability, but some scientists believe that free radical production is important to the development of endurance training adaptations.

Another interesting area of recent research concerns the use of probiotic drinks to improve intestinal health and reduce the risk of developing the common cold. Probiotics are thought to lessen (but not eliminate) the risk of developing an upper respiratory tract infection by reducing the amount of disease-causing bacteria in the intestinal tract. Several well-controlled studies of endurance athletes have provided provisional support for these claims. However, more research is required before the use of probiotics can be confidently recommended to assist immune system function in rowers and other endurance athletes.

TRAINING SUGGESTION #6: INCREASE PROTEIN INTAKE WHEN TRYING TO LOSE WEIGHT

Most indoor rowers do not need extra protein, especially when body weight is stable and they consume normal amounts of meat and dairy produce. However, indoor rowers who are attempting to lose weight by reducing daily caloric intake may benefit from a relative increase in dietary protein. A daily protein intake of between 0.8 and 1.2g per kg of body weight (approximately 10–15 per cent of total energy intake) is usually considered appropriate for good health. Increasing relative protein to between 1.2 and 2.0g per kg of body weight (approximately 15–25 per cent of total energy intake) can improve appetite control due to its greater satiating effects when compared to fat or carbohydrate. This can make it slightly easier to control hunger sensations and improve adherence to dietary targets. If an increase in daily protein is desired, consider eating more protein rich foods such as meats, fish and eggs as well as vegetarian options such as soya, nuts and seeds.

Increased protein intake may also be able to attenuate the loss of fat free tissue (including skeletal muscle) which normally accompanies weight loss. Approximately 75 per cent of the total weight loss from successful diet or aerobic exercise interventions is due to loss of fat tissue, while the remaining 25 per cent comes from loss of fat free tissue. Since 2000m rowing performance is related to the total fat free mass of the rower, it is particularly important to try and minimise the loss of fat free mass when attempting weight loss. A modest increase in dietary protein has been suggested as one way to help improve fat free mass preservation. One way to increase protein intake is to consume milk after rowing training. In fact, a study conducted at McMaster University in Canada found that ingesting 500–1000ml of skimmed milk (bovine) shortly after resistance training was able to produce a simultaneous increase in fat free tissue and decrease in fat tissue in young women who performed resistance training. Whether similar benefits occur after aerobic training and when attempting weight loss is presently unclear, but post-exercise milk ingestion has other well-established benefits which include enhanced rehydration, immune boosting effects and carbohydrate replenishment. Also, milk and other dairy produce can make an important contribution to bone health, and evidence is accumulating that links the incidence of stress fractures in lightweight rowers with reduced bone mineral content. An increase in dietary protein, including extra dairy intake, may be especially helpful to the health and rowing performance of lightweight competitors when actively attempting to reduce body weight.

TRAINING SUGGESTION #7: SELECT HEALTHY FOOD CHOICES WHICH ARE ENJOYABLE

Supermarkets provide an extensive and diverse range of healthy food choices but, in practice, many people actually only select from a very small range of foods. This narrow approach to shopping reduces the need for conscious consideration of food choices and makes it easy to just put the food in the basket and get past the checkout desk as quickly as possible. If you allow yourself a little more time in the supermarket to take a more diverse look at the foods on offer, especially in the fruit and vegetable and fresh food sections, you may find switching toward a better balanced diet much easier. Keep in mind that any healthy change to your usual shopping routine will need to be sustainable in order to gain the full health benefits. Consider the following suggestions to improve your chances of making healthy and sustainable food selections:

- Avoid shopping during peak times or when you are hungry or tired.
- Take a prepared shopping list which includes several healthy choice items that you don't normally purchase (e.g. dried fruit, low fat sauces, unusual fruits or vegetables, frozen fruits and vegetables, soups, fresh pasta and noodles, stir fry mixes).
- Read food labels and try to get a better awareness of the energy content and proportions of fat, carbohydrate and protein (occasionally try to guess what a food label might say before looking).
- Select the healthier versions for some of your usual items (e.g. reduced salt and low fat versions of the same food).

- Reduce the number of high-fat and high-sugar foods for purchase or select smaller pack sizes.
- Reduce the number of prepared 'ready' meals that you purchase and instead try to make similar meals from the fresh ingredients.
- Consider purchasing a range of non-perishable sports foods which can be stored in your training bag or car. These can be available for consumption before or after training (e.g. carbohydrate/protein bars, gels and beans).

TRAINING SUGGESTION #8: AVOID TRAINING ON AN EMPTY STOMACH

Indoor rowers often fail to eat appropriately before training and frequently underperform as a result. Some rowers worry that eating too close to a rowing session will make them ill. This is especially a problem for early morning rowers who train soon after waking. Some indoor rowers think that training adaptations are better when training is performed in a fasted state. Often, rowers end up training on an empty stomach just because they fail to plan meal times carefully. Alternatively, the entire training session may be skipped because an indoor rower only recognises their hunger at just the moment that they need to make a conscious decision to go to training, electing instead to eat rather than exercise. Irrespective of the reasons, training on an empty stomach can decrease enjoyment and reduce training quality.

The standard recommendations for pre-exercise food intake state that a carbohydrate rich and low fat meal should be consumed at least 3 hours before the start of training. There is actually no reason to avoid eating a carbohydrate rich meal closer to the start of training. The 3 hour target that is often quoted was largely based on the preferences of athletes, especially distance runners. It is acceptable to eat food right up until the beginning of a session, but common sense suggests that it would be prudent to select smaller portion sizes to reduce the chance of stomach upset. It is also a good idea to avoid consuming large quantities of food near the start of a high intensity rowing session to avoid gastric reflux.

Indoor rowers can experiment with food timing before typical training sessions to discover what suits their personal preferences or better yet, set out a clear plan to eat well in advance of training. Most modern mobile phones allow a user to programme an electronic reminder at set times on set days. Some indoor rowers, particularly those with busy daily schedules, may find it helpful to set up weekly reminders to eat approximately 3 hours before usual exercise times.

Liquid-based carbohydrate meals (e.g. yogurt drinks) are particularly good before an early morning session, as are a range of other cereal based snacks or fruits. Select low fat foods that provide at least 50g of easily digested carbohydrate along with an appropriate amount of fluid. Possible examples include:

- 2 cereal bars
- 300ml fruit smoothie
- 250g of baked beans on toast
- Chocolate bar (standard size)
- 700ml of a sports drink
- 2 bananas or 3 apples
- 1 or 2 sports bars/energy bars (50g per bar)
- 1 or 2 packets of jelly beans or similar confectionary (30g per pack)

TRAINING SUGGESTION #9: PRIORITISE TOTAL ENERGY INTAKE WHEN TRYING TO INCREASE FAT FREE MASS, BUT DON'T FORGET ABOUT PROTEIN TIMING

Plenty of competitive indoor rowers want to increase body weight through the addition of muscle mass. Providing that the gain in muscle mass is confined to the muscles that are important for indoor rowing, increasing total muscle mass and body weight can often improve 2000m performance. There are two points of special importance for indoor rowers who want to increase fat free mass. First, for significant gains in fat free mass to occur (>2.0 kg) it is usually necessary to include weight lifting as a regular part of training (typically three sessions per week for eight weeks or more). Second, it is necessary to develop and maintain a positive energy balance by increasing daily energy intake by 500 to 750kcal.

The source of the additional energy is less important than often suggested, but it is advisable to provide most of the additional calories from carbohydrate and protein rich sources to keep body fat gains to a minimum. It is worth noting, however, that the increase in muscle mass from weight lifting is enhanced when 10–20g of essential amino acids are consumed soon after weight training. This can be achieved by consuming standard foods (e.g. two to four eggs, 200–400g of low fat yoghurt or 200–400g of baked beans) or using sports supplements (e.g. 20–40g of whey protein). Consuming 500–1000ml of bovine milk (skimmed, semi-skimmed or full fat) is probably the best and cheapest option to help indoor rowers meet the targets for both essential amino acids and total energy intake.

If there is little change in body weight and fat free mass after eight weeks of appropriate weight training, then a stricter approach to ensuring a daily energy surplus on all days of the week may be needed. Strategies that may help develop a suitable and sustained positive energy balance can include any of the following ideas:

- Eat more frequently rather than trying to eat several large meals.
- Increase the use of high energy, low fat snacks such as creamed rice, fig rolls and liquid meal supplements.
- Limit the intake of bulky foods that are high in fibre (e.g. enriched cereals and breads).
- Prepare meals in advance (freeze if required) to improve the amount and immediate availability of food soon after training.
- Seek assistance from a qualified sports nutritionist and complete a full dietary profile to better assess energy requirements.

Making weight for lightweight indoor racing

Indoor races typically offer a lightweight category for men and women in each age category starting at Junior 18. The maximum permitted weight for men is 75kg (165lb) and 61kg (135lb) for women. Competitors are required to weigh in on the official competition scales and have their weight certified by an official between 1 and 2 hours before the scheduled race time. The inclusion of lightweight events across most age divisions at major indoor regattas has helped develop indoor rowing into a major sport. Nevertheless, many lightweight competitors struggle to make the weight limits in time for competition, usually due to inexperience or poor nutrition in the days before competition. At least lightweight rowers who fail to reach the maximum permitted weight cut-offs are usually still allowed to race in the openweight competition, but they often underperform due to the earlier effects of trying to make weight.

> The maximum permitted weight for men in lightweight competition is 75kg (165lb) and 61kg (135lb) for women.

Racing in a lightweight category is very appealing to many individuals, especially for rowers whose normal body weight is slightly higher than the maximum permitted weight. In the extreme, a few indoor male and female competitors have attempted to lose as much as 10kg or more to make weight. With enough time, careful planning and a good deal of willpower it is possible for some rowers to achieve these large reductions in body weight. However, indoor rowers should consider the likely effects on health and performance before attempting significant amounts of weight loss. Indoor rowers who have healthy body fat levels when they begin weight loss (e.g. 15 per cent for males and 25 per cent for females) often report slower 2000m ergometer performances once the target body weight has been achieved, despite many weeks of hard training. This finding is partly explained by the loss in total fat free weight that usually accompanies reductions in body fat. Furthermore, the expected physiological gains from training are often reduced, and possibly eliminated, when a rower is engaged in a period of sustained negative energy balance.

It has also been reported that immune function and bone mineral content are adversely affected when healthy individuals attempt significant amounts of weight loss. Rowers increase their risk of developing injury, illness and infection during periods of weight loss and nutritionists typically advise that weight loss should be achieved gradually over prolonged periods of many weeks to minimise these risks. Nutritionists also suggest that the majority of the weight loss target should be achieved well in advance of the competition date. In practice, this is still relatively rare and lightweight competitors who need to lose weight typically do so over the final four weeks before a major event. As with other complex nutrition problems, indoor rowers who are considering a substantial reduction in body weight should first consult a well-qualified sports nutritionist to establish the relative safety of their ambition and to discuss possible nutrition and training strategies that minimise the potential for health complications and performance loss.

Making weight immediately before competition

Analysis of the weight making strategies used by top jockeys, wrestlers, boxers and rowers has revealed that food and especially fluid restriction are the preferred choices of athletes who need to reduce body mass in a short time period. Perhaps unsurprisingly, as rowers become more experienced at making weight, the amount of weight loss successfully achieved in the final week before competition increases slightly. It is common for male and female lightweight rowers to achieve target weight after losing between 1 and 2kg in the previous 7 days. These losses are achieved by reducing energy stores, typically from fat and carbohydrate reserves, along with a

relatively minor loss of body water. Ideally, it would be better for reasons of convenience and avoidance of health risks if lightweight rowers were able to successfully weigh in at their natural body weights. Nevertheless, the available information, both from research and anecdotal experience, suggests that top lightweight competitors routinely manipulate their body weight in the days before a major competition. In fact, top competitors report that their 'normal' body weights are usually several kilograms above the maximum limits for competitive racing. Given that most rowers will reduce their body weight in the final days before a competition, at a time when training is relatively light due to the need to rest before competition, dietary strategies are likely to be of considerable importance. Thus, indoor rowers need to develop food and fluid intake strategies that allow for the necessary weight loss to be achieved while avoiding any potential loss in rowing performance.

Guidelines for making weight safely for indoor rowing competitions
General
- Avoid excessive or rapid weight loss; fat free mass is better preserved when large weight losses (>4 kg) are achieved over seven weeks rather than four weeks or less.
- Target a daily energy deficit of 500kcal to achieve a weekly weight loss of approximately 0.5kg.
- Consider having your body composition measured at regular intervals to monitor fat free mass and fat mass changes.

- Avoid extreme dietary practices during training, especially low carbohydrate or high fat diets.
- Consider an increase in relative protein intake, especially through milk and dairy produce intake.
- Practise weight loss and weight recovery strategies well in advance of competition.

Pre-competition

- Limit weight loss in the final 24 hours before competition to no more than 5 per cent of normal body weight.
- Fluid restriction can be used in the final 12 hours before competition, but limit dehydration to a maximum of 2 per cent of body weight to allow opportunity to restore fluid deficit post weigh-in.
- Avoid carbohydrate loading; a carbohydrate intake of 5g per kilogram of body weight is suitable on the day before a 2000m competition.
- If weight targets allow, eat a light carbohydrate rich meal (approximately 50g) approximately 3 hours before competition.
- Avoid use of laxatives or appetite suppressants.
- Avoid use of steam rooms, saunas or rubber suits.
- Additional weight loss can be achieved with moderate intensity exercise.
- Consider the use of a low residue diet for 24 hours before competition (e.g. minimise intake of whole grain products and high fibre food).

Post weigh-in

- Avoid eating beyond comfort levels.
- Avoid binge eating soon after weighing in, especially large quantities of solid food.
- Liquid meals, sports drinks and small snacks are the best food choices.
- Salty snacks or the addition of small amounts of salt to a sports drink can help restore fluid deficits due to dehydration.

NUTRITIONAL SUPPLEMENTS FOR INDOOR ROWING PERFORMANCE

Nutrition supplements are products that claim to have health benefits or performance enhancing effects when taken in addition to a person's typical diet. The popularity of nutrition supplements is apparent in the growing number of dedicated health food shops that sell various potions and pills to help manage a range of health issues including joint aches, memory loss, gastrointestinal problems, stress, sleep loss and skin problems. Supplements are also popular with athletes. Surveys suggest that between 60 and 90 per cent of elite athletes in a range of sports regularly consume one or more nutritional supplements. The most popular choices are vitamin and mineral supplements but caffeine, creatine and various amino acid supplements are also widely consumed. There is a common perception among athletes that taking specific supplements will aid performance and improve the ability to cope with high training volumes.

The decision to use nutrition supplements is not one to take lightly. Rowers should be especially cautious about the range of exaggerated manufacturer claims displayed on product labels, as well as the high risk of consuming a product that contains unsafe ingredients. Many products simply cannot live up to the claims on the label and there is good evidence to show that approximately 5–30 per cent of sports supplements available for purchase in a selection of countries (including Germany, Australia, the United Kingdom, the United States and South Africa) can produce a failed drugs test when used as directed by the manufacturer. For example, several commercial weight gain products were found to contain anabolic steroids or prohormones, neither of which were stated on the list of ingredients. While this may have been the result of poor manufacturing practice and ineffective quality control, there is also isolated evidence of manufacturers deliberately adding banned or illegal substances in an attempt to enhance the reputation of their product as an effective aid to performance. The typical consumer is usually unaware that the sale of nutrition supplements in most countries is controlled by food and drink laws rather than the much stricter laws which apply to medicines and medical claims. Furthermore, the agencies responsible for monitoring a supplement manufacturer's claims, as well as assessing the supplement ingredients, are limited in their capacity to respond to the vast number of products currently available for public consumption. Indoor rowers who are planning to use nutrition supplements should exercise considerable caution before making any purchases.

It is extremely easy to buy nutritional supplements. Health shops, sports shops, online stores and even supermarkets all offer a wide variety of products at reasonably affordable prices. Of the diverse range of products targeted at consumers interested in sporting performance, most will typically claim to improve muscle strength, muscle size, physical endurance or mental alertness. Unsurprisingly, products that make claims about their ability to reduce body fat are especially numerous. While there are specific ingredients which scientists have shown beyond reasonable doubt to improve the physiological response to exercise, the actual number of effective ingredients is small. Most indoor rowers will gain far greater health and performance benefits from making improvements to the quality of their normal daily diet rather than investing in supplements that may have limited effectiveness. Several nutrition supplements, however, can make reasonable claims to improve indoor rowing performance. Such claims are justified by the results of published scientific research which has been independently reviewed and approved by nutrition experts.

The following nutrition supplements may provide worthwhile benefits to indoor rowers during training and racing:

- Caffeine
- Creatine
- Beta-Alanine
- Sodium bicarbonate (or other alkaline salts such as sodium citrate)

These supplements are widely available in general food stores and specialist retailers and their use is not prohibited by the 2011 World Anti-Doping Agency (WADA) guidelines. The next section describes further details about each of the four supplements including the typical supplementation patterns. Key findings from studies that included a measure of ergometer rowing performance are detailed. Importantly, the possible mechanism(s) of action which may help explain performance effects are also discussed. There are other supplements which have less scientific data to support their efficacy, however, it is not possible to provide an exhaustive list of such products and indoor rowers should consult a well-qualified sport nutritionist before deciding to use such products.

CAFFEINE

Caffeine is a popular stimulant found in chocolate, soft drinks, tea and coffee and is widely sold in pill form at service stations and university campus stores. It has multiple effects on the body and is known to alter the availability of various hormones and neurotransmitters. Until 2004, caffeine ingestion above a moderate intake level (typically around 200–400mg) was banned by the International Olympic Committee (IOC) due to the likelihood that it would give an unfair advantage to users. However, various studies at this time had suggested that the full performance enhancing effect of caffeine could be achieved at intake levels below the threshold needed to fail a drugs test. Thus, taking higher doses of caffeine only increased the risk of failing a drugs test without providing any additional benefits to performance. Experts also recognised that the widespread popularity of caffeine-containing foods, drinks and medicines would make an outright ban on caffeine impractical. Caffeine is deliberately consumed by many athletes and is generally considered to be both a legally permitted and effective performance enhancing substance for use in a range of sports.

Are there benefits to taking a caffeine supplement?

Many studies have confirmed the benefits of caffeine consumption for a variety of sports. Benefits have been demonstrated for brief high intensity events such as sprint cycling, middle distance running as well as prolonged cycling and running tasks that last several hours. Caffeine was originally believed to improve endurance performance by increasing the use of fat stores to fuel exercise. Greater use of fat stores could reduce the reliance on the body's limited reserves of carbohydrate, enabling an athlete to maintain a slightly faster pace before reaching the point of fatigue. However, researchers have struggled to detect a consistent effect on fat utilisation and this proposed mechanism could not explain caffeine's ergogenic (i.e. performance enhancing) benefits during events of less than 90 minutes, where fatigue is unlikely to be caused by carbohydrate depletion. Caffeine has even been shown to improve the performance of cyclists during events lasting as little as 1 minute. Researchers have yet to provide a complete explanation for caffeine's performance enhancing effects, but the most likely reason is that caffeine acts on the brain to reduce the perception of fatigue and decrease pain sensations, possibly by stimulating greater release of endorphins or by blocking pain receptors.

Several well-controlled research studies have provided strong evidence that caffeine can increase 2000m ergometer rowing performance in both male and female rowers. For example, researchers at the Melbourne Institute of Technology investigated the effect of giving trained male rowers different amounts of caffeine or a placebo 1 hour before completing a 2000m test on a Concept2 ergometer. On three different days, rowers drank a solution which contained either 0, 6 or 9mg of caffeine per kilogram of body mass. Average performance time was approximately 1 per cent faster when caffeine was ingested in comparison with the placebo trial (412 seconds to 416 seconds, respectively). Although caffeine improved ergometer performance, there was no added benefit to consuming the higher amount of caffeine (9mg/kg). These researchers repeated the study with female rowers and again found that both the 6mg/kg and 9mg/kg doses of caffeine improved 2000m ergometer performance in comparison with a placebo. However, the average improvement in performance time was slightly better when the 9mg/kg dose was ingested (~1.3 per cent faster than placebo) than when the 6mg/kg/dose was ingested (~0.7 per cent faster than placebo). Analysis of the 500m splits suggested that the improvement in 2000m performance time was largely due to a faster opening 500m section.

One of the difficulties in making use of the results from the Melbourne studies is the relatively large amount of caffeine required to gain a performance benefit. For example, a 70kg rower would need to consume a total of 420mg of caffeine at the lower recommended dose of 6mg/kg 1 hour before competition. While this amount of caffeine would not be considered excessive by regular drinkers of strong coffee, it is still far more than most people's daily caffeine intake. Caffeine also has well-known mood altering effects and can increase anxiety and irritability, something which is particularly undesirable shortly before an indoor rowing competition where anxiety levels are usually very high already. More recently, researchers have suggested that performance in a

range of sports can be improved by ingestion of smaller amounts of caffeine, even as little as 1 to 3mg/kg.

While caffeine use appears to be an effective way to improve rowing performance, it should be noted that not all researchers report a clear improvement in rowing performance. Researchers in Queensland (Australia) failed to find any significant differences in 2000m rowing ergometer performance when trained oarsmen ingested 0, 2, 4 or 6mg/kg of caffeine 1 hour before exercise. One important difference in this study was that the rowers consumed a light meal shortly before ingesting the caffeine which appears to have decreased the rate of caffeine absorption. These researchers also noticed that while some rowers appeared to receive a performance benefit from caffeine, other rowers did not. The extent to which caffeine is ergogenic for an indoor rower is likely to be affected by their tolerance and sensitivity to caffeine. It may still be possible for highly sensitive individuals to benefit from caffeine if lower doses are used or tolerance is built up over time.

Potential side-effects of caffeine

Side effects, if present, are usually minor and short lasting and may include increased anxiety, muscle tremor, gastrointestinal upset, headaches and possible alterations to heart rate.

Caffeine is generally well-tolerated when consumed in doses of 1 to 9mg/kg by otherwise healthy individuals. The usual doses of caffeine needed to achieve an ergogenic benefit are similar to the amounts of caffeine routinely ingested by drinkers of brewed coffee from commercial outlets. However, most studies to date have provided caffeine in a powder or pill form and it is not entirely clear if the performance enhancing effects are altered when caffeine is ingested in popular drinks. Indoor rowers who wish to use caffeine to improve race performance should first experiment with different intake strategies during training to check for potential side effects and to decide if caffeine is helpful for them. It is worth noting that caffeine is a popular mood enhancer and may increase motivation to exercise which could also improve training adherence.

CREATINE

Creatine is a non-essential nutrient which is stored in muscles as the high energy compound phosphocreatine. Regular consumers of meat are likely to have a modest intake of creatine since red meat and fish such as tuna and salmon are popular sources of creatine. The human body can also manufacture creatine from other sources of protein, so individuals who have a restricted intake (e.g. vegetarians) will still have some creatine in their muscles. However, creatine stores are typically lower in vegetarians than in individuals who consume a mixed diet, which suggests that the body cannot manufacture creatine in sufficient quantities to offset a low dietary intake. There are no known health risks to having low creatine levels but there are performance implications for individuals who participate in very high intensity exercise such as sprinting, weight lifting and jumping.

The energy for muscle contraction is provided by the high energy compound ATP. The amount of ATP stored in the muscle is miniscule and requires rapid replenishment by one of several biochemical pathways within the muscle. The pathway which provides the highest rate of ATP provision relies on the energy generated from the splitting of stored phosphocreatine to synthesise ATP. Importantly, the production of ATP from phosphocreatine does not depend on the availability of oxygen. However, the body's stores of phosphocreatine are very small and reach critically low levels after only 30 seconds of maximal exercise. While this might seem rather unimportant at first, this pathway provides ATP as soon as exercise starts and provides enough time for other ATP-generating pathways, particularly those that rely on the availability of oxygen, to reach peak rates of energy production.

Various studies over the last 20 years have shown that daily supplementation with 5–25g of creatine per day for up to four weeks (usually in the form of creatine monohydrate) is effective for increasing the muscle's phosphocreatine stores by approximately 20 per cent. The increase in phosphocreatine should extend the amount of time that the muscles can produce ATP at very high rates, both through elevated energy stores and by improving the muscle's ability to buffer lactic acid.

Are there benefits to taking a creatine supplement?

While there are good reasons to think that an increase in muscle phosphocreatine after dietary supplementation should enhance 2000m ergometer performance, it must be remembered that anaerobic energy sources only supply approximately 20–30 per cent of the energy needs of a 2000m race and the phosphocreatine stores only contribute part of the total anaerobic energy supply. At best, the improvement in 2000m ergometer performance from the typical ~20 per cent increase in stored phosphocreatine is likely to be a matter of only a few seconds.

Researchers at Birmingham University provided the first strong evidence that creatine monohydrate supplementation can increase ergometer rowing performance. Two separate groups of trained male and female rowers were matched according to sex, body weight and 1000m indoor rowing performance. On each of 5 consecutive days, one group received creatine monohydrate dissolved in a flavoured drink (~10–20g/day depending on body size) while the other group received the flavoured drink only (control group). Neither the subjects nor the experimenters knew who was receiving the supplemented drinks. The 1000m ergometer performance was measured immediately before and after the 5 days. Average performance was unchanged in the control group at 214 seconds before and after the 5 days. However, subjects in the creatine monohydrate group improved their 1000m ergometer times from an average of 211 to 209 seconds. The researchers were also able to show that the performance improvements were linked to the amount of creatine retained by each individual. The subjects who retained the most creatine after supplementation (indicated by low amounts of creatine in urine) were also more likely to experience improved performance than subjects who were less able to retain the ingested creatine. Since this study measured 1000m performance, which has a higher anaerobic energy requirement than 2000m, it would be helpful to know if creatine supplementation might also enhance performance over the standard race distance.

The combined effects of training and creatine supplementation on 2000m ergometer rowing performance was addressed by research conducted at The University of Alberta in Canada. Scientists compared the ergometer performances of students before and after six weeks of training (~35km/week of ergometer rowing and two sessions/week of resistance training). Each day, the experimental group received flavoured drinks which contained dissolved creatine monohydrate (15–30g per day for the first 5 days before intake was reduced to 1.5–3 g per day for five weeks) while the control group received the same drink but without creatine. Both groups achieved impressive training gains: 2000m times improved by an average of 18 seconds in the creatine supplemented group and by 15 seconds in the placebo group. However, by the strict statistical rules of scientific research there were no differences between the groups for change in 2000m performance. The researchers also made note of how hard the two groups were training during the six week study since one of the popular suggestions for the benefits of creatine is that it allows users to train harder. However, there was no evidence in this study that the creatine group was performing either the ergometer interval sessions or the resistance training any harder than the control group. The researchers concluded that creatine supplementation did not improve training response or improvements in 2000m ergometer rowing performance after six weeks of standard training. Unfortunately, the researchers used a mix of rowers and non-rowers in both groups and it is likely that the very large improvements in 2000m performance after only six weeks of training were due to a combination of improvements in rowing technique and low initial fitness. Given that the effect of creatine supplementation on athletic performance and training capacity is likely to be very small, any potential benefits of creatine are likely to have been hidden by the much larger overall changes in technique and fitness of these subjects.

After 20 years of intensive research, creatine supplementation is now well established as an ergogenic aid for sports which require explosive, high intensity bursts of energy (e.g. weight lifting and sprinting). However, the improvements in performance are relatively small and appear to be highly specific to each individual. Indeed, some individuals fail to gain any increase in the amount of creatine stored in their muscles. Research studies where samples of muscle tissue have been extracted and analysed for creatine concentration before and after creatine monohydrate supplementation have revealed an upper limit to the amount of creatine that can be stored. Individuals who begin a period of supplementation with low initial levels of muscle creatine typically experience the greatest increases in stored creatine, whereas individuals who have high initial levels may not experience any change in stored amounts. This is one reason why vegetarians tend to respond better to creatine supplementation than non-vegetarians. Researchers have also discovered that the increase in intramuscular creatine stores are enhanced when extra carbohydrate is consumed during the supplementation period.

There are good reasons to believe that creatine supplementation may be helpful to competitive indoor rowers seeking to enhance 2000m performance, however, the benefits are likely to be small. Indoor rowers who are successful at increasing intramuscular creatine stores are likely to be able to train marginally harder during high intensity training activities (e.g. resistance training or repeated bursts of high rate rowing). There are also reasons to be cautious about the use of creatine, especially for lightweight indoor rowers. One of the clearest indications that a person is increasing intramuscular creatine at the start of supplementation is a significant gain in body weight, usually between 0.5 and 3.0kg in the first week. The increase in body weight is simply due to a transient fall in urine output and subsequent increase in fluid retention. Weight gain does not reflect changes in muscle protein, although some of the retained fluid will cause swelling in the muscles. Some researchers have speculated that this muscle swelling provides an important stimulus for muscle growth (hypertrophy) after training periods of six weeks or more. Nevertheless, the extra total body fluid will increase the energy cost of body movements during indoor rowing and makes it more difficult for lightweight rowers to manage their body weight targets. Rowers who wish to try creatine supplementation to see if it benefits their training and competition should do so early in the season and monitor changes in both body weight and high intensity indoor rowing performance.

> It typically takes up to 1 month to restore normal body weight once creatine supplementation is discontinued.

BETA-ALANINE

The amino-acid beta-alanine has gained popularity with many indoor rowers for its potential to improve indoor rowing performance. It is found in meat and fish and is also widely sold in powder or capsule form. Beta-alanine is essential for the manufacture of another protein, carnosine, which can act as both an anti-oxidant and as a pH buffer. It has been suggested that beta-alanine supplements can increase carnosine concentrations in the skeletal muscle and increase acid buffering capacity. Potentially, indoor rowing performance may be enhanced if supplementation with beta-alanine is able to increase muscle carnosine levels and provide a meaningful increase in muscle buffering capacity.

Scientists at Ghent University (Belgium) reported that rowing ergometer performance over a range of distances (100m, 500m, 2000m and 6000m) was greatest for trained rowers who possessed the highest amounts of muscle carnosine. Next, the scientists ranked the rowers according to their 2000m performance and then randomly allocated individuals of similar ability into either a control group (placebo) or an experimental group. Rowers in the control group received a placebo, while rowers in the experimental group consumed 5g per day of beta-alanine. After seven weeks of standard training, the rowers were re-tested for muscle carnosine content and 2000m ergometer performance. There was a 35 per cent increase in lower leg carnosine content for the beta-alanine group, but no difference in the control group. The change in 2000m performance after the training period tended to follow the changes in muscle carnosine levels. Before supplementation, both groups had an average 2000m performance of 6:30. After supplementation, the beta-alanine group had improved by 2.7 seconds, whereas the control group had slowed by 1.8 seconds. This suggests that the combination of rowing training and beta-alanine supplementation may provide a benefit of just over 4 seconds. These provisional results need to be confirmed by other researchers, but it does appear that beta-alanine supplementation may be an effective way to improve 2000m ergometer rowing performance.

SODIUM BICARBONATE (ALKALINE LOADING)

High intensity rowing substantially increases the production of lactic acid inside the active muscles and the subsequent release of hydrogen ions increases muscle acidity. It is the hydrogen ions that stimulate free nerve endings insides muscles, causing the painful sensation commonly experienced during intense exercise. Once the hydrogen ions have been produced, they are quickly buffered by chemicals and proteins within the muscle, or released into the blood, where additional buffering agents are present. Researchers at Ohio University conducted a novel experiment to discover the pattern of lactic acid production during ergometer rowing. Trained rowers first completed a maximal 6 minute ergometer test, after which a researcher obtained a blood sample to measure the lactate concentration. On a subsequent occasion, the same rowers repeated the 6 minute ergometer test, matching their pacing profile from the first test. This time, however, the researchers stopped each rower at specific time points (either 1,2,3,4 or 5 minutes after the start) and measured the blood lactate concentration. These concentrations were then directly compared against the lactic acid concentration measured at the end of the 6 minute test on the first day. This research design allowed the researchers to provide evidence that lactic acid is rapidly produced in the rower's muscles within the first minute of a simulated competitive effort. In fact, it is likely that most of the lactic acid produced during a 2000m ergometer test is formed within the first minute, requiring rowers to perform at maximal effort despite a high level of muscle acidity. Eventually, the acidity overwhelms pain receptors inside the active muscles and sends an electrical signal to the brain to stop rowing.

While interval training still presents the best solution to guarding against high muscle acidity, nutrition strategies that increase the blood's buffering capability may slightly delay the onset of fatigue during a 2000m ergometer race. Sodium bicarbonate (baking soda) has been used with some success by indoor rowers. It has also been used successfully by on-water rowers in Olympic competition. The results of a number of research studies suggest that a dose of between 100 and 300mg/kg body weight is optimal when ingested 1–2 hours before exercise. The sodium bicarbonate is usually dissolved in 500 to 1000ml of flavoured water. These studies generally provide evidence for small benefits to exercise performance during high intensity events lasting between 1 and 7 minutes. There is limited published evidence concerning the use of sodium bicarbonate for indoor rowing performance. One Australian study reported a small but significant increase in the distance completed during a 6 minute maximal effort on a Concept2 rowing machine with a 300mg/kg body weight dose. However, the study only involved a total of five well-trained oarsmen which is too small a sample to make meaningful conclusions. Recommendations regarding the effective use of sodium bicarbonate for 2000m indoor rowing performance rely heavily on the results of non-rowing studies.

The major problem with sodium bicarbonate use is the high risk of uncomfortable side effects. These include diarrhoea, bloating, cramps, gastrointestinal discomfort and vomiting. In fact, most indoor rowers who have tried sodium bicarbonate loading will have experienced many of these side effects. It does appear to be possible to reduce the side effects by consuming additional amounts of fluid along with the sodium bicarbonate. There are also suggestions that spreading the dosage over the 24 hour period before exercise can achieve similar performance benefits with a much reduced risk of side effects.

Researchers have also tried to use sodium citrate as an alternative to sodium bicarbonate to further reduce side effects. The effective dosage required for sodium citrate use is typically between 300 and 500mg/kg body weight.

SPORT NUTRITION IN THE 21ST CENTURY

Recent advances in the scientific study of sport and exercise nutrition have substantially improved understanding of the role that food and drink play in determining training responses. Scientists are now focussing particular attention on the relationship between diet and specific physiological adaptations to training. By studying the genetic basis for training adaptations, scientists are beginning to isolate the cellular signals responsible for increasing muscle size or building mitochondria. Clearly, the extent to which a person can benefit from endurance training, as well as the rate at which they make physiological changes, is substantially controlled by genetic inheritance. While we cannot change our parents, it is possible to use nutrition interventions to change the way that our genes function in order to improve sports performance. This research is gathering pace and it is likely that the results of these studies will contribute plenty of new ways to use nutrition to improve future indoor rowing performance across all ability levels.

Summary

Nutrition supplements can be used to enhance indoor rowing performance when ingested shortly before a 2000m race (e.g. caffeine and sodium bicarbonate) or in the days and weeks before a race (creatine and beta-alanine). The performance gains are typically very small and only in the order of a few seconds. These amounts may be of considerable benefit to top indoor competitors in the open categories, where an improvement of even just a few seconds can mean the difference between victory and finishing outside the medal positions. However, performance gains from supplementation are not guaranteed and indoor rowers may have to cope with some uncomfortable side effects. All indoor rowers who are considering the use of nutrition supplements should try different loading protocols and examine the possible benefits during training and certainly well in advance of a major competition. For most indoor rowers, the largest gains in rowing performance are likely to come from achieving suitable fluid and energy intakes before and during training.

// CASE STUDIES

10

The aim of this chapter is to provide information about the experience of a number of successful indoor rowers. There are also two case studies that portray the development of rowing in schools.

ANNA BAILEY

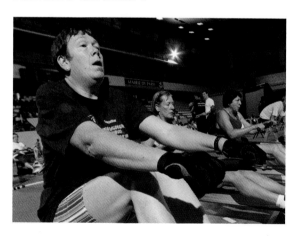

Anna Bailey is one of the most successful indoor rowers in the UK. She is the current World Record holder for 2000metres in the 50–54 (and therefore 50–59) age category, a record she set in 2001. She has won the British Indoor Rowing Championship nine times and the World Championship five times. She still also holds every 50+ world record

from 1 minute to 100km, and will move into the 60–64 age group in January 2011.

Before moving into indoor rowing Anna was a keen squash player and had also been successful at netball, hockey and tennis. She describes herself as needing to be good at whatever she does – a hallmark of top athletes.

Indoor rowing began for Anna in 1999 with a cold call from her local gym inviting her to become a member. After trying various types of equipment, Anna felt most at home on the rowing machine – and took part in a challenge to row 10km in under 45 minutes – something she thought was impossible. However, with some training she soon went under this time and also won £1000 for a 2km competition within the chain of gyms she was a member of. This led her to compare her times with those published on the Internet, which is when she realised that she had the potential to compete at the top level. She won Bronze in the 2000 World Championship and Gold in 2001. Since then she has been the top woman indoor rower in her age group.

Anna looks back in horror at her first experience in the gym on a rowing machine. The assumption was that because she was strong, the damper setting should be on 10 and the instruction she received was rudimentary (she now rows with a drag factor of 125). Even now she sees beginners in the gym being taught badly – and she finds it difficult not to intervene. Anna was fortunate to find an excellent coach in Eddie Fletcher who taught her a technique very similar to that of rowing on water.

'The differences are that we (indoor rowers) keep the chain straighter but we aim for the same flowing movement. We row alongside mirrors a lot so that we can check our posture at different points in the stroke'. Anna likes the friendliness of the indoor rowing community: 'We help each other a lot with technique and training tips. After a race, no one asks about your placing; they ask "How was it for you?" It's all about your individual performance against the machine.'

At times Anna has felt pressured to achieve and it has been her fellow competitors who have helped her to maintain a sense of perspective.

> Indoor rowers are very friendly – there will always be some one willing to offer help and advice.

Anna tried rowing on water but did not find the same sense of camaraderie. 'Also, it was frustrating waiting for crews to be sorted out – and noting that some people were very choosy about who they rowed with. As a new person in a crew, I was made to feel that I was the one causing the problems.' In contrast, Anna can train on her ergo in her own time, with her own music and at a level of intensity that suits her.

At times motivation to train can be a problem. 'I have my ups and downs, and at times I can hardly bear to go near an ergo. My coach is very supportive and tells me to do something short and simple. I find that doing my pre-race warm-up routine helps to get me over this feeling. When I'm on an up it's great. I've been known to get up at 4 a.m. to put the hours in. These days I tend to train after work. Injuries can be a problem although I did compete in Denmark with a broken wrist by rowing one-handed.' Anna's wish is that she could motivate herself better!

Nervousness before a race is still a problem for Anna. 'Like most people I spend a lot of time in the toilet but going through my 20 minute pre-race warm-up routine calms the nerves and enables me to go out and do the job.'

Anna's advice to anyone thinking about becoming involved in indoor rowing is: 'Find a good instructor; too many gym instructors know little about developing good technique. Go to small local competitions and meet up with people who will help and support you. Beware of online forums; there is no way of knowing what the quality of the advice is – and some of it is dangerous. As you begin to develop, find yourself a good coach.' And finally: 'Training has to be fun.'

GRAHAM BENTON

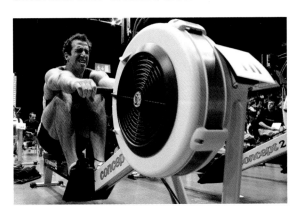

The early years of the BIRC were dominated by international rowers such as Steve Redgrave and Matthew Pinsent. It was thought that the superior rowing technique learned on the water would make the top rowers unbeatable on the ergometer. When Graham Benton, a non-rower, won the Men's Open category in 2004, it sent shock waves around the rowing community. The reaction was that this must have been a 'one-off event'. However, Graham went on to win the same event in 2005, 2006, 2007, 2008 and 2010. After winning the Men's World Championship in the 30–39 age group in 2004 and 2005, he became the Open World Champion in 2006.

From the age of 11 through to 30 Graham's main sport was cricket. He played for his county and for Welsh Schools as a teenager, and more recently for Havant Cricket Club, one of the top club sides in the country. From his mid teens Graham had been a member of a gym but mainly used weights to maintain and build up strength rather than as cardiovascular workout.

At the age of 21 his gym ran a 500m ergometer competition. 'I did a 1:19. At the time I knew it was quick for my gym but had no idea how quick it was in the bigger scheme of things so it wasn't until when I was 29 that my then gym, Roko in Portsmouth, had a 2000m competition. It was probably after that race when I started to believe that I was something more than average on the ergo. I gradually whittled my time down from 6:35 to 6:09 without really knowing what I was doing. The South of England Indoor Rowing Champs were a few weeks later and I entered and came second to Nik Fleming in 6:03. From that point I was pretty much hooked and was training every weekday to try and be the fastest non-rower ever.'

Graham gradually developed his own technique: 'I had a rough idea about what felt efficient and strong so just worked on keeping pressure on the handle for as long as possible. I coached myself based on what got my split down. I was aware that I wanted a strong consistent stroke so always worked on low rate, steady training. I did used to set a mirror up in the early days as well.'

His initial training sessions were self-planned: 'I would sit on the rowing machine and do what I fancied. I always worked hard, maybe too hard, but it was a lot of sprint work rather than long-distance structured training. I had help with a few sessions from a guy called Chris Hetherington who was probably my first coach and then after I'd shown a fair degree of promise and wanted to take it to the next level, I started working with Eddie Fletcher who is a long time indoor rowing coach and well respected on the scene. Eddie has looked after me whenever I have needed it for the past five years or so.'

Graham's main focus for training is now rowing on water but he still trains about 12–15 hours per week – a mixture of water sessions, weights, cycling and the ergometer. He found the transition to rowing in boats challenging and is full of admiration for the way in which good rowers make the action look so easy. However, training is not a problem: 'I have always loved training. The racing, on the ergo or the water, is something that is always in the back of my mind and keeps me at it. I'm very good at making myself train even if I really really don't want to and it is the thought of the British Indoors Championships and the pressure to perform, or the desire to win Henley, that keeps me going. I do think if I wasn't competing I would still train though, perhaps not quite as hard and probably more focussed on specific things that are more enjoyable. I love trying to improve which is one reason why I bought a Watt Bike [a static exercise bike] as it was a way I could keep training interesting as there would be a whole new set of personal bests (PBs) and records to aim for.'

His advice on training is: 'If you are genuinely committed and motivated, then you will still train barring some sort of major reason. I tend to work on training bands – so if I know I have had a really hard day or I know my mentality is not good, then I set myself a slightly more achievable target. It's amazing how often you end up beating that target in the end but at least it gave you the confidence to do the training session. It's not about PB-ing every day or constantly improving. It's about training at approximately the right intensity for a certain time, so don't get too upset if your 16k ergo is 2 seconds slower than last week as you have still done 16k training and that is in the bank. Take advantage of your good days but don't beat yourself up too badly on your off days. It's about trends over months and years, not day to day. My training tips would be get a goal, plan a structured training programme to achieve it and stick to that programme. Get in the routine of doing what the programme states whether you feel in the mood or not. Once you start missing sessions without a damn good reason then it's a slippery slope.'

Graham gives a great deal of credit to his coach Eddie Fletcher: 'Eddie Fletcher has been absolutely key to me hitting the scores year after year. Eddie brought consistency to my training and from that I developed a belief and an understanding of almost exactly what I was capable of at any given time. I think that trust in Eddie and my training is the thing that has enabled me to push on through the middle of races when my mind might be telling me otherwise.'

For someone with as much success and experience as Graham, pre-race nerves are still a problem: 'I really struggle with pre-race nerves. I get nervous every time I have an ergo test. I try and have a routine. I will sometimes have a little book where I write a few bullet points to remind me of what I am capable of. It will list some key sessions that I have nailed in the previous weeks, some of my key achievements, a few inspirational statements, etc. I am literally a bag of nerves almost every time, though, until the machine says "Row" and then I tend to slip into what I know I can do. I think the key thing is knowing your capabilities and believing in your training. If you trust your training, then regardless of how much it hurts you know that you can carry on.'

Graham's advice to future champions is: 'Go for it. I have constantly had to reset my goals as I kept achieving them. I thought I could just slip under 6 minutes and did that easily. I got down to 5:51 and won the 30–39 Worlds and thought that was as good as it would get. I remember thinking I will never go faster than that. I wanted to win the British Indoors and did that, six times now. And got down to 5:42, which was beyond my wildest dreams. I know I have been in good enough form at times to go quicker than that too but haven't delivered on that form when it mattered. And winning the Open Worlds was amazing. So I'd say don't underestimate your capabilities and do everything you can to give yourself the best chance to realise them. There are plenty of people willing to give you advice, some good and some bad. Watch how the best people operate and adapt what they do to work for you. Nik Fleming was my main inspiration and role model to begin with. I saw him as relentless in his training, and he thrived off being the best. Other people's admiration brought out the best in him.'

TERRY COGING

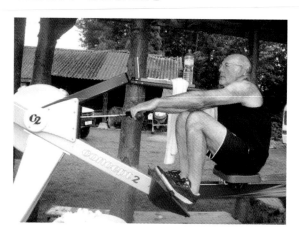

Terry Coging is the 2010 British Champion in the over 70 age group. Terry's first sport is cycling – indoor rowing is something he does as a sideline or when he has been injured. In fact, he won the BIRC while recovering from eye surgery. Terry suffered from a detached retina when he was 28 and, on medical advice, gave up cycling. The operation in 2010 was a success and enabled Terry to see properly for the first time in years.

Terry had a few successes in cycling between the ages of 16 and 27 but then had a long break until returning to the sport at 55. By this time Terry was totally deaf, which made racing in groups too dangerous, so he transferred to time trials. He started winning veterans events (including national championships) throughout his sixties. He still holds the 12 hour distance

records from when he was 61 and 62 (262 and 260 miles!). Two crashes put an end to his racing career – and he had a new hip fitted at 66. Unfortunately, after the operation, Terry was unable to get his trunk into a good enough position for bike racing as he was too upright – but he was able to use an ergometer.

Terry had first used an ergometer at the age of 58 to augment his training for cycling in the winter. He was having back problems at the time and using the ergometer seemed to help – so he bought his own.

Terry does not consider himself to be a top indoor rower, simply 'Blessed with a good engine.' In fact, a good cardiovascular system is a prerequisite for success in most power sports. Terry has never trained for more than 16 weeks – and in fact lives for part of each year in France without access to an ergo. He has also had long breaks due to operations. In spite of this, the monitor on his 5-year-old Concept2 is reading 3500km. 'There has not been much doing on the bike, so I have to do something.'

In terms of technique, Terry is self-taught, and has never received any coaching: 'But I read a lot and have studied videos.' His training has been based on the Pete Plan (http://thepeteplan. wordpress.com/the-pete-plan/) and he is good at listening to his own body. His motivation for training is 'To keep in good nick ready for cycling in the springtime,' although Terry does admit to training seriously for the British Championships. He believes strongly that 'Training must be regular and involve sufficient rest.'

For 40 years Terry has not added salt, sugar or butter to food – and eats lots of fruit and vegetables – but otherwise eats anything.

His advice to any ex-cyclists or people from other sports who are considering converting to indoor rowing is: 'Read a lot and question everything. And, as Herb Elliott said, enthusiasm gets you started but habit keeps you going.' His advice for race preparation is: 'Start a week before and practice visualising the race. Do a well planned and practised warm-up and have absolute faith in your training.'

DEBBIE FLOOD

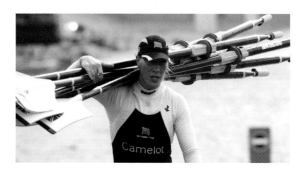

Debbie's sporting career began when she joined in fun runs with her dad at a very early age. Running was her first love and she went on to represent Yorkshire Schools at 1500m and cross-country

Debbie's achievements

The chronological list of Debbie's achievements is long and impressive:

1997	British Indoor Rowing Championship (BIRC) Junior Championship, Gold Medal
1998	World Indoor Rowing Junior Championship, Gold Medal
1998	World Junior Rowing Championship, Bronze Medal (with Frances Houghton)
1999	World U23 World Championship, Gold Medal (with Frances Houghton)
2000	World Rowing Championship, Women's U23, Gold Medal (in a single scull)
2002	Winner of the World Cup Rowing Championship (with Frances Houghton)
2003	BIRC Women's Open, Gold Medal
2004	Olympics, Women's Quad, Silver Medal
2005	World Cup at Lucerne, Bronze Medal (with Elise Laverick)
2006	Winner of the World Cup Rowing Series with two Golds and one Silver
2006	World Rowing Championship, Women's Quad, Gold Meda
2007	Winner of the World Cup Rowing series with two Golds and one Silver
2007	World Rowing Championship, Women's Quad, Gold Medal
2008	Olympics, Women's Quad, Silver Medal
2009	BIRC Women's Open, Gold Medal
2010	BIRC Women's Open, Gold Medal
2010	World Rowing Championship, Women's Quad, Gold Medal

(and also the shot putt). Because her journey to and from school often involved passing through a rough area, Debbie took self-defence classes. Her natural sporting talent and competitive spirit soon resulted in her becoming a member of the British Junior Judo Squad. At about this time Debbie's dad, who was still running, injured his knee and began to use an ergometer as part of his rehabilitation programme – and naturally, Debbie gave it a try as well. Within a short time she was posting remarkable times and was encouraged to enter the 1997 British Indoor Rowing Championship, where she won the Women's Junior event.

As a result of this win Debbie was encouraged to try rowing on water. Although she found the transition difficult, she worked hard and was soon doing well enough to have to choose between judo and rowing. In the end it was not a difficult decision: 'Alec Hodges at Tideway Scullers School was so friendly and encouraging. I dreamed of going to the Olympics and being good enough to represent my country so I gave rowing a go to see if I would get anywhere. I then enjoyed it so much and loved the people I met who accepted me and believed in me, so much so that they kept me going through the times I wasn't doing so well.' It was around this time that another rowing coach told Debbie that it was unlikely that she would ever be more than a 'competent club rower'. Fortunately, Debbie decided to prove him wrong.

By 1998 Debbie was a member of the GB Junior Squad and was heading for the World Junior Rowing Championships, where she won a Bronze Medal with Frances Houghton in a double. In spite of being a popular member of the squad, Debbie describes herself as 'having started as an outsider' as the majority of the members in the Junior Squad had come from prestigious rowing schools. Now the popularity of the sport has increased, senior squad members come from varied backgrounds around the country. Debbie still speaks with a soft Yorkshire accent and is proud of her northern background.

As well as the annual list of impressive results in both rowing on the water and indoor rowing, and the training required to achieve these, Debbie also attended Reading University and graduated in 2005 with a degree in Physiology and Biochemistry.

After the Beijing Olympics in 2008 and 11 years of full-time training, Debbie decided to take an 18-month break to qualify as a prison officer. During this time she only trained once or twice a week with a view to returning to full-time training and winning a place in a crew boat for the 2012 Olympics. Her ultimate career aim is to work with young offenders.

For many rowers the ergometer is an instrument of torture, an experience to be endured – but not for Debbie: 'I relish ergo tests because I want to know how well I am doing. During training sessions on the ergo I'm always counting, for example, I listen to music tracks; I know the length of each one and how far that should take me. Alternatively I set a rate and only count the strokes that are exactly on the rate. If I'm racing, I know what split times I need to achieve so I concentrate on maintaining them. I can't let my mind wander or I would lose my posture and risk injury. Racing at an indoor rowing event is much tougher than rowing on the water. On the water things are constantly changing and it takes your mind off the pain. On the ergo it is simply a matter of counting down the metres.'

Debbie's training on the ergometer is part of a fixed schedule for the GB Squad – she never has time to prepare specifically for indoor rowing events. 'Motivation makes a big difference to training. Our main motivation is our end goal, and that for us is winning an Olympic Gold Medal – that is good motivation to train hard! But day in day out it's not as easy as that and there are days when you don't feel like training and you are extremely tired! But we know that every training session counts. Medals are won and lost by fractions of seconds and each training session makes a difference. We also have a great team environment and we all go through down times at some stage so we help each other and encourage each other.'

Debbie's advice to anyone who is struggling to improve is: 'Hard work will lead to improvement. That's how it works. It may be baby steps or giant leaps, it may take weeks, it may take years, but the thing is to focus on your personal improvements and making yourself better and stronger by training. There will be ups and downs as in anything. It's never all smooth but it's about achieving your potential and if you have worked hard to do that then you can be proud whatever the result.'

In spite of all her achievements, Debbie still needs strategies to cope with nerves: 'Race prep starts well before race day – knowing that you have trained well and hard and are looking forward to racing. Everyone is very different but I like to be calm and relaxed and confident right up 'till the last minute, then before I boat to race or go into the indoor ring I use aggression to get myself ready and the adrenaline that naturally comes with nerves. When I first started racing I would be so nervous that my knees would be shaking at the start, but as the years have gone by I have learned to control that and, although I still get nervous, I am outwardly calm so nobody would ever know how nervous I am.'

> Training is about achieving your potential, and if you have worked hard to do that, then you can be proud whatever the result.

Throughout her rowing career Debbie has always made herself available to talk to groups in schools and community centres. Her enthusiasm, warm personality and achievements have provided an example and inspiration for hundreds of young people.

ROBIN GIBBONS

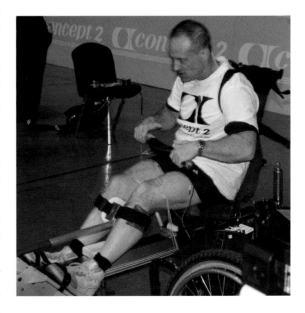

Robin Gibbons is a former navy diver and commercial airline pilot with Virgin Atlantic. In 2001 a car accident left him paralysed from the waist down.

Following his accident and long recovery, Robin took up swimming in order to get the cardio-vascular exercise he needed to prevent the increased risk of developing the so-called diseases of inactivity, such as coronary heart disease, that people with a spinal cord injury (SCI) are prone to develop. However, his research into the subject showed that the majority of people with an SCI are unable to voluntarily exercise enough muscle mass to gain optimal exercise benefits. He also realised that although swimming fulfilled an appropriate volume of exercise, it was not intense enough, so he began to look for alternatives.

Robin believes that 'When you search for solutions, you create opportunities.' The opportunity came when in March 2003 he saw a demonstration of Functional Electrical Stimulation (FES) rowing at the London Regatta Centre.

FES was developed nearly 30 years ago at the University of Alberta in Canada. FES uses very small electrical impulses to stimulate the nerves that supply paralysed muscle groups and, in so doing, initiate muscle contraction. By supplying these impulses through electrodes placed in strategic places on the surface of the skin, paralysed limbs can be made to move. A microprocessor in the stimulator can be programmed to automatic sequencing of leg movement, or when coupled to a simple switch, control of the legs during rowing for example.

What Robin saw seven years ago was one of the first demonstrations of FES rowing which had been developed by Professor Brian Andrews while working in Steadward Centre at the University of Alberta, Canada. The team have researched the use of FES as part of wider research into reducing common health problems suffered by people with an SCI.

Robin described the first FES rowing machines as 'Looking very agricultural!' However, the machine did provide the opportunity for the level of cardiovascular exercise that Robin was looking for 'because this enabled a person with an SCI to exercise using all four limbs', so he joined the project.

With his technical background, Robin was able to contribute to improvements in the design of the system. For example, while the legs are able to extend to drive the seat back, their inability to fully flex to return the seat back to catch meant that bungy cords had to be used to assist. Robin had the idea of using gravity by inclining the FES-rower. This resulted in the back of the rowing machine being raised so that gravity can be used to return the seat unit back to the catch: 'I thought about the ramp at the end of an aircraft carrier flight deck and reversed the effect.'

In November 2004 Robin Gibbons and Sol Solomou competed in the first FES rowing competition at the BIRC. This was recognised by the presentation of special medals to Robin and Sol by the Olympic Gold Medallist, James Cracknell.

Robin established world records three years running in the 2km FES category which was eventually beaten by the Paralympic Gold Medallist Tom Aggar in 2006. He is very keen that the 2km distance remains even though the international adaptive events on water are 1km. Robin is now able to sustain work rates for 30 minutes that previously he could only sustain for some 12 minutes three years ago.

In 2008 Robin embarked on a PhD studentship to investigate cardiorespiratory adaptations to an FES rowing programme. Robin's studies have included designing an appropriate FES rowing exercise programme to enable an accurate assessment of the changes in cardiovascular fitness. Although Robin has some two to three years to go before completing his doctorate, he explains, 'We need reliable evidence to prove the benefits that FES rowing can offer. To date we have achieved oxygen consumptions of almost 3 litres of oxygen per minute – a level associated with the non-disabled population.'

> FES rowing is not just about competing, it's about providing the opportunity to exercise and avoid illness.

Robin believes that a commercially available system for home use is still a long way off: 'One of the problems is establishing an organisation responsible for this unique type of training. Because of this it is more likely to be conducted by specialist training centres around the country.' In talking to Robin it is obvious that he is frustrated by the slow progress in making FES more widely available. He is, however, optimistic about future developments. 'If we develop eight channel systems in place of the current four channel one, we can stimulate the gluteus maximus and the gastrocnemius muscles to increase the ability of the legs to flex, which will have a dramatic impact on the metabolic demand and as such cardiorespiratory health.'

Robin's advice to anyone interested in FES rowing is 'Contact me at robin.gibbons@virgin. net'.

DAVE HOLBY

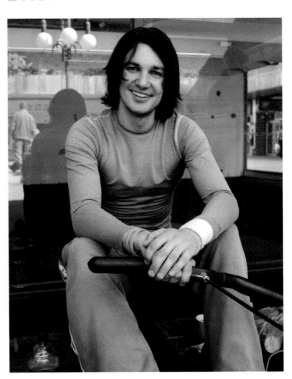

Dave Holby, an actor, is arguably the 'world record-holder of world records for indoor rowing' – he holds eight of them. Dave took up conventional rowing at the age of 15 after being inspired by Steve Redgrave's fourth Olympic Gold Medal in the 1996 games in Atlanta. He continued rowing at Exeter University and competed at the British Universities Sports Association Championship and at Henley. 'I was one of the lightest guys in the boat so I was always stuck in the bow seat – but I loved it.'

Fund raising with a rowing machine followed in his final year when, with a friend, he undertook sponsored rows in a number of city centres and also collected money from members of the public.

While on an acting job in Birmingham he had the idea for a longer fund raising row with the objective of raising money for Breakthrough Breast Cancer. After Google searches on the length of The Great Wall of China (too short) and the distance to the Moon (too long), he settled on the circumference of the Earth at the equator, a distance of 40,075km. Discussions with the Guinness Book of Records resulted in the granting of a new world record category – but with a specification of 300km per week. Dave chose Basingstoke town centre as the venue for his record attempt but hit a problem. Street collections are licensed by the day, rather than for 5 days a week for a period of two and a half years. However he did manage to negotiate support for the project on the basis of a three-month rolling licence. Concept2 also supported the project with the gift of a new machine. So on May 28, 2008, Dave set off around the world on a rowing machine. He made it more interesting by plotting a route of the target distance that linked cities of the major continents. Following his progress between countries and cities became a major project for many local school children, who also supported him in the town centre.

To meet the specification for a new world record, Dave had to row an average of 60km for 5 days each week. 'The first two weeks were tough but I gradually settled into it, although one of the problems was managing to eat enough calories. I started off weighing 76kg and dropped to 66kg in the first month.' Dave found that he needed to maintain an intake of 6000kcal per day. He also managed to maintain his career as an actor but had to make up the 300km weekly average when work took him away from

his rowing machine in the the town centre. DIY work in the evenings was also a requirement to earn his keep.

On December 18, 2010 Dave completed the 40,075km to establish a new world record as well as raising over £20,000 for Breakthrough Breast Cancer. During the two and a half year period, he also broke seven other world records.

> To break world records you need the support of a team of friends and family.

So what was the motivation? 'Well, there were many dark days when it was so difficult to get up facing the prospect of yet another day of 60km on the ergometer. What got me through it was the support of family, friends and the hundreds of supporters who came to see me rowing. They were not going to give up on me – and this provided the motivation to keep going.'

Also for Dave it was not only a virtual journey but also a real journey of self-discovery. 'I found out a lot about myself, what I could do, what I was capable of, and I met so many fantastic people who gave me their support and friendship.'

Dave's advice for anyone attempting to break any of his records is: 'You need a support team of friends and family who will be with you every stroke.'

1   100km tandem rowing world record – with Dave's brother, Jonathan in a time of 7 hours, 31 minutes
2   24 hour tandem rowing world record – with James Burrows, a combined distance of 312.7km

3   Million metre rowing world record – lightweight world record for fastest million metre row, time 227 hours, 43 minutes

4   Endurance rowing world record – lightweight world record for endurance rowing of 30 hours

5   Greatest metres rowed in a season record – 17,111,960m

6   Million metre tandem rowing world record – with Ollie Trinder, time of 102 hours, 32 minutes

7   Endurance tandem rowing world record – with Ollie Trinder, in 103 hours

8   Fastest time rowing around the equator (40,075km) in 934 days

GEOFF KNIGHT

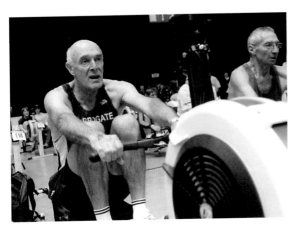

Geoff Knight holds the world record for lightweight men in the 70–74 age group in a time of 7 minutes and 13.4 seconds. To put this in context, it is almost two seconds faster than the British open (i.e. heavyweight) record for the same age group, and very close to the Open World Record. This is an outstanding achievement for some one who weighs less than 75 kg.

Geoff has competed in every British Championship since 1992 when he won a Silver medal in the 50–59 age group. Since then he has notched up a total of 10 Golds and 4 Silvers.

Like many successful indoor rowers, Geoff played other sports before turning to indoor rowing. He played amateur rugby league before switching to Rugby Union during his period of national service. He retired from playing rugby at the age of 40 and took up running, completing a total of 8 marathons and numerous cross country and fell races. However, in 1991 Geoff developed a knee problem and joined a gym to keep fit until it recovered. 'I became hooked on the ergometer immediately I found I was fairly good.' Although Geoff began with a need to maintain fitness whilst nursing an injury, he discovered that it was the best form of all round exercise he had tried, and one that provided him with some goals to achieve.

Geoff has never received much coaching. He uses information from the Concept2 website about technique and training. 'From January to July I train 3 x 1 hours per week with several breaks for holidays (I am retired with a wife and a caravan). From July to September I train 4 x 1 hours per week with fewer breaks. From September to the British Championships in November, I train 5 x 1 hours per week and try to avoid any breaks. The training is based on the training guide plus weight training if I feel up to it.'

For Geoff, it is the competitions that provide the motivation to train: 'Indoor rowing would be fairly boring without a target which the BIRC provides'.

On the subject of diet: 'I don't follow a special diet but just eat a lot of what I'm told is good for me. I enjoy most foods but don't eat much red meat and seem to be able to eat lots of sweet stuff without exceeding the lightweight limit. I found it easier to maintain my stamina when I was able to both run and row.

Geoff must be one of the few people in this world who does not suffer from pre-race nerves: 'I try to keep moving before an event but others prepare in different ways and I think everyone must find what works for them. If I have trained successfully in terms of attaining the times and distances set in the training guide, I know that if I row to my plan I should hit my target. However, I know from experience that I cannot row as fast in training as I can in competition so I never row the 2000m distance in training.

Geoff's tips for anyone keen to become involved in indoor rowing: 'Join a gym – it provides a useful social dimension' and a heart monitor is 'invaluable in measuring progress and providing you with reassurance when the red mist descends'. Geoff describes the 'red mist' in terms of the state he often experiences in the last 500 metres of a 2000 metre race when the conscious perception of things begins to recede. At this point, he relies on the information from the heart rate monitor to continue: 'I believe that the body can be pushed to a level well outside its comfort zone and that the heart monitor can provide some reassurance when the body is sending out signals to slow down.'

GILL PRESCOTT

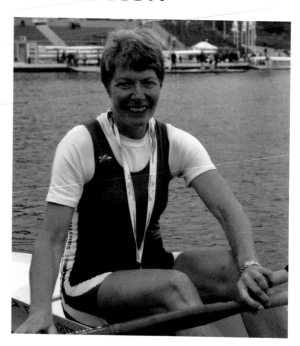

In 2005 Gill Prescott, a veterinary surgeon with three children (triplets), joined Durham Amateur Rowing Club to learn to row. By 2006 she had won a Gold Medal at the BIRC in the 45–49 age group. In 2007 she became the European Champion (50–59) and in 2008 the World Champion (50–54) – and had won several major regattas in a quad. In 2008 Gill also took second place in a single at the the World Veteran's (now Master's) Championship. She was the British National Indoor Rowing Champion in her division from 2006–2010. In 2011 she is heading the world rankings and has no intention of giving up yet! This is an astonishing rate of development and achievement.

Before taking up rowing Gill's main sporting interest was running – and she still runs every day as part of her training routine. She considers herself lucky to have met Geoff Graham, a coach at Durham Amateur Rowing Club, who spotted her potential as an indoor rower and encouraged her to enter competitions. Since 2005 Geoff has been her coach both on the water and on an ergo. In spite of a busy professional and family life, Gill has enjoyed competing: 'It has been so much fun going to all of these competitions.'

For some people competitions provide the motivation to train. Not so for Gill – she loves the training and competitions are a bonus! She trains every day except Thursdays – and often twice a day if work allows. The training includes running and rowing both on the water and on the ergo. 'The ergo is a great way to get fit but I prefer to be out on the water.'

Since suffering stress fractures of the ribs Gill has included weight training in her routine – which she believes keeps her free from injury. Her training regime is based on the Concept2 plan, but modified to suit her life and work. Her recommendation is to train alongside others (and a good coach): 'Training does hurt and my times are never as good when I'm training in the garage by myself. Having a good coach does help with the motivation.'

Gill still gets very nervous before competitions, and like others, uses her warm-up routine to focus: 'Once the race starts, I really enjoy it.' Her advice to indoor rowers: 'You can learn something from every race.'

APPENDICES

1 PLANNING A SERIES OF COACHING SESSIONS

It is important to begin with an overview of the sessions and the main objective to be achieved. A planning grid is an essential tool for this purpose. For example, the main objective for a group of young beginners might be:

After five sessions of 90 minutes you should be able to exercise on the rowing machine using a technique that will maximise your effort, your enjoyment and reduce the chances of strain or injury.

Key words: kinetic chain, pushing with the legs, drive phase, recovery phase, relaxation, rhythm, ratio, catch, finish.

Sample training plan

Time in minutes	Week 1	Week 2	Week 3	Week 4	Week 5
5	• Introductions • Safety procedures	Review of week 1 objectives	Review of week 2 objectives	Review of week 3 objectives	Review of week 4 objectives
10	Icebreaker activity (see p. 30)	Repeat of week 1 activities	Repeat of week 2 activities	Warm-up exercises	Repeat of week 4 activities
5	Objectives and demonstration	Repeat of week 1 activities	Repeat of week 2 activities	Repeat of week 3 activities	Repeat of week 4 activities
15	Activity 1 in pairs – in turn on ergo pushing back (no handle, no display)	Separation of drive and recovery phases: concept of ratio	Use of the display to check the rate	Repeat of week 3 activities	Introduction to simple training plans and web-based resources
5	Explanation and demo of the kinetic chain	Practical activity on ratio	Practice maintaining slow rates	Use of the display for split times	Introduction to competitions
15	In pairs, pushing back with the legs holding the handle with arms straight leaning forward	Practical activity on ratio	Rowing at rating 20 maintaining good posture	Rowing to a constant split time	Relay competition in teams – rate capped at 20

Sample training plan *(continued)*

Time in minutes	Week 1	Week 2	Week 3	Week 4	Week 5
15	In pairs, swing back at the finish drawing handle into the body	Rowing together using rhythm and ratio	Rowing together following a leader	Following a leader rowing to a split time	Repeat, but aiming to maintain good posture
5	Review and feedback	Review and feedback	Review and feedback	Review and feedback	Review and feedback
15	In pairs, putting the stroke together in slow motion	Feeling power during the drive phase	Warming down exercises	Improving power in the drive phase, plus warm down	Attempt PBs over 500m, plus warm down
10	• Review of key points • Objectives for next session	• Review of key points • Objectives for next session	• Review of key points • Objectives for next session	• Review of key points • Objectives for next session	• Review of course • Celebrate success!

A planning grid for a group of adults with little experience of exercise would be signifi-cantly different. The main objectives and the steps towards achieving this need to be tailored to the group, the resources and the time available.

Working in pairs helps to develop a 'buddy' system in which each rower can check on the other to ensure good posture – or any signs of discomfort or distress such as gasping for air or facial expressions showing extreme pain.

Individual session plans include sub divisions of the main objective into 'bite-sized chunks'. For example, the objectives for session 1 in the example above might be:

By the end of the session the participants should be able to:

- point to the safety exits and know where the assembly point is;
- draw the attention to the coach of anyone who appears to be uncomfortable or in distress;

- explain what a kinetic chain is – and why it is important in terms of posture when using the rowing machine;
- demonstrate that rowing is more of a pushing than a pulling sport; and
- name the basic parts of the rowing machine – and clean it at the end of the session.

A key part of the planning process is to review each session in terms of the responses of the participants, what you did that worked well, or what you said or whether you did not achieve the results you expected and what you need to do differently next time. There also needs to be flexibility within each session as you respond to individual needs and limitations.

PROGRESS AND SELF-ASSESSMENT FORMS
Self-assessment sheet
This is an example of a self-assessment sheet that can be used by participants to check their own

progress, and also as a basis for a discussion with the coach. The form is for you to assess and record your own progress using the numbered criteria below. It also provides a basis for the questions that you need to ask. Discuss your self-assessment with your coach.

1   I haven't a clue. Will someone please explain this again from the beginning.

2   I think I understand but would benefit from a further explanation.

3   I'm getting there and I know when things are going well.

4   I can feel how I'm improving and I now know what I need to do to improve.

5   I'm feeling confident on this aspect and I know what I have to work on.

Learning outcomes for the first five sessions of using the rowing machine

At the end of the following sessions you should be able to:

Experimental group

Level achieved

| | 1 | 2 | 3 | 4 | 5 |

Session 1

Identify the emergency exits and know the procedure in the event of an emergency

Observe how the technique used on the ergo might be different from the styles you have seen in gyms

Explain the importance of a kinetic chain in terms of a sequence of movements

Observe others and identify some basic errors such as sitting upright or pulling with the arms

Feel the effect of pushing with the legs as the main source of power

Identify what you hope to get out of rowing

Identify the main parts of the ergo and know how to clean it at the end of a session

Session 2

Understand the differences between the drive phase and the recovery phase

Row taking more time during the recovery phase (e.g. in a three or four beat count)

Understand the importance of relaxing the shoulders and arms in the recovery phase

Identify good posture at the catch and finish

Know the importance of wearing appropriate clothing for the conditions

Row in synchronicity with others experiencing good rhythm and ratio

Begin to feel that you can apply power through the legs

Session 3

Understand the basic functions of the display and drag lever

Row maintaining a steady reading on the strokes per minute function on the monitor

Follow a leader so that you row at the same rate and rhythm

Improve your posture at the catch and finish positions

Develop a good sequence of arms, body legs throughout the stroke

Develop more confidence in applying power in the drive phase

Session 4

Understand the importance of warming up and warming down

Row maintaining a steady reading on the split time for 500m function on the monitor

Apply pressure through the legs while maintaining good posture

Identify common faults in posture and technique

Use mirrors and posters to check your own posture and technique

Session 5

Understand the basic principles of training – and the importance of rest and recuperation

Know where you can find resources to help you with a training plan

Review your aims in learning to use an ergometer

Establish your personal best time (PB) for 500m

Experience some competition

Identify what you need to work on to improve your posture and technique

Know how to make training fun

Assessment for coaches

As a coach you should be seeking feedback both from the participants in your sessions and other coaches who are willing to observe you in action. This is a form you could develop for your own use. Remember to leave space for comments. Use the following numbered criteria:

1 Excellent – clear evidence provided of appropriate professional behaviour

2 Good – some minor aspects to consider

3 Satisfactory – but give careful considerations to the comments below

4 Unsatisfactory – this is an aspect that you need to improve on

5 Weak or non-existent – you need to seek help and support with this aspect of your coaching

Assessment of coaching sessions

The coach:	5	4	3	2	1
1 Identify the emergency exits and know the procedure in the event of an emergency					
2 Provided in advance an outline plan of the sessions showing how this fits in to an overall programme					
3 Established a safe, positive and friendly learning environment					
4 Explained/reinforced how to achieve good posture and technique – and why it is important					
5 Was clear and concise when giving instructions					
6 Asked questions in a way that reinforced understanding					
7 Was fair and equable in dealing with all participants					
8 Provided challenges that were appropriate to the group and individual members					
9 Gave summaries of learning points at appropriate times					
10 Provided an appropriate amount of input during the session					
11 Provided appropriate feedback during the session in a warm, encouraging and inclusive manner					
12 Made good use of voice communication in terms of appropriate variation of pace, pitch and projection					
13 Knew the name of each participant					
14 De-briefed the participants with a summary of what had been achieved by eliciting comment and feedback from the participants					
15 Encouraged participants to take appropriate responsibility for cleaning and checking equipment					
16 Outlined targets for the following session					
17 Ended sessions on time and on a high note					

2 ROWING IN SCHOOLS
GET GOING GET ROWING

The Get Going Get Rowing project is based in the northeast of England, and so far has involved over 18,000 children in 70 different schools. The project is a partnership between the Tony Blair Sports Foundation (TBSF), Concept2, British Rowing, Competition Managers, NHS North East and Sport Universities North East England (SUNEE).

TBSF was launched in 2007 with the aim of involving and improving the health of the region through sustained investment in local people to inspire them to make the most of themselves through sport. In particular, the foundation aims to build capacity by training new coaches from within the local community. Indoor rowing is one of the six sports that has been selected for this kind of support.

In partnership with Concept2, TBSF raised funds for 90 rowing machines so that more schools in the region could have sufficient machines to establish a Northeast Indoor Rowing Competition. The local strategic health authority began to fund the competitions on the basis that exercise provides significant health benefits for both adults and children. The Senior Competition Managers, TBSF and SUNEE worked in partnership with British Rowing to establish the competitive pathway which was trialled in the school year 2008/2009. This pathway is based on a series of steps beginning with intra-school then inter-school events (including virtual leagues) right through to county finals and culminating in a northeast regional final. The first Get Going Get Rowing northeast regional final took place on March 2, 2010 and involved the best 192 athletes from County Durham, Northumberland, Tees Valley and Tyne & Wear.

The following were key elements to ensure success:

- The recruitment and funding of 39 volunteers committed to the project, who took the British Rowing Level 1 Indoor Rowing Coaching Qualification
- The training, by British Rowing, of competition managers, school sport coordinators and teachers
- The provision of an information pack to participating schools
- The loan of Concept2 machines
- Excellent promotion and publicity to ensure participation and wider interest
- Support from local rowing clubs to schools without rowing machines
- A dedicated core team of organisers

The promotional work included:

- The production of a promotional DVD featuring Olympic Gold Medallist and TV presenter James Cracknell
- Free promotion through the websites of British Rowing and Concept2
- Excellent publicity through local radio, TV and newspapers

The role of the main partners has been crucial in developing an inclusive competition structure that enables both established rowers and those new to the sport to take part. The event has been promoted through the established network of School Sports Partnerships – groups of schools working together to develop physical education and sport opportunities for all young people.

From the beginning the emphasis has been on establishing a sustainable development programme that will embed indoor rowing as a sport in local schools. Already there is evidence that this is happening, and local rowing clubs have experienced a growth in membership.

For anyone thinking of developing a similar project in their region, the organising team have the following advice:

- Have a clear vision of how you see the structure developing and expanding.
- Get the buy-in from key partners to ensure sustainability and growth.
- Establish links with clubs early on to provide an outlet for those individuals who are attracted to the sport and help clubs find and train volunteers to support this growth.
- Be prepared for enjoyment and success!

LONDON YOUTH ROWING

In the London borough of Brixton young people who are part of a gang culture do not venture into Hackney as it is 'enemy territory'. Likewise, Brixton is off limits to Hackney gangs – or rather it was until indoor rowing came to town, enabling members of youth clubs in these areas to compete on ergometers over the Internet and to realise that they have more in common than they thought.

These events, and much more, are organised by London Youth Rowing (LYR), a charitable organisation founded in 2004 by Jim Downing, an American and ex-city banker. Jim had seen community rowing in action in the United States and wondered why, after seeing the exclusive nature of rowing in the UK, there was nothing

similar to offer young people in inner cities. So he approached London Youth, The Federation of London Youth Clubs with 70,000 members spread over 400 clubs, and the London Regatta Centre in Newham, East London, which provided services mainly to schools. This scheme had very limited success because all of the facilities were based in one centre.

The next step was to obtain funding from the MAN Group, sponsors of the MAN Booker Prize and a world-leading investment group. The MAN Group funded LYR for five years, providing funds to set up the organisation and the development of projects and initiatives. A further agreement was between LYR and Concept2 who saw the possibilities of the idea and supported this project with the loan of 80 machines. These were placed in schools, youth clubs and community groups predominantly in East London and allowed for the development of wider usage and locally based competitions, but there was still only limited success in the uptake of the project.

The breakthrough came with the appointment of Matt Rostron. Matt had been involved with Hollingworth Lake Rowing Club in Lancashire and in developing indoor rowing competitions, to the point that we now have the English Indoor Rowing Championships and a re-launched Regatta At The Club. Matt and two colleagues realised that more support and publicity was required to ensure that the ergometers in schools were fully utilised. In partnership with Sport England and private funders they gained a further £1.4 million to establish Row East London, and to place five ergometers in 50 per cent of the schools in East London. Part of the deal was that the school signed up to a 'contract' of joint objectives that included setting up an indoor rowing club, training for staff, collection of registers and data and participation in competitions. Within a short time the Row East London project had five community coaches, each supporting development in approximately 15 secondary schools (or two London boroughs) each. The project team developed teaching resources aimed at making the experience of indoor rowing fun – and to enable the teachers to manage classes of up to 35 students with only five ergometers in a single session.

Promotion was still needed to get the message across that 'Indoor rowing is here to stay.' As part of the marketing strategy, Matt and his team offered taster events across the whole of Greater London, including on the runway of City Airport. A key message was that schools could have access to indoor rowing within their own schools and clubs. A key factor was that Matt and his team were flexible and quick to make changes in response to the needs of different groups. Through development events for the London Youth Games, they were able to established a high profile for indoor rowing in all 33 London boroughs.

There is now a competition structure in place between the London boroughs. LYR, in partnership with London Youth Games, also organises three events: the Indoor Rowing and Adaptive Events and also the On-water Regatta. They also launched the National Junior Indoor Rowing Championship, which has become one of the largest or indoor rowing events in the world. In 2010 there were over 3000 entries, more than in the World Indoor Rowing Championship held every year in the United States. Matt stresses the importance of making these events fun for young people to attend: 'As well as the rowing there are lots of other cool activities such as a climbing wall, graffiti boards, skateboarding and brush boarding/ surfing – these make it a fun day and make the young people want to come and compete in future years.

London Youth Rowing is not limited to indoor rowing. The team sees the need for pathways to rowing on water – inevitably participants eventually ask the question: 'We've done the indoor rowing, what now?'

LYR offers the chance to learn to row at 11 sites across London, and they also run the junior section at three clubs, where they provide coaching and support to the existing club structure. There are also organised Learn to Row courses which are run five times per year for six weeks at a time. From these courses there is a 55 per cent conversion to club membership in West London and a 33 per cent conversion rate in East London. This is considerably higher than from most Learn to Row courses.

They also offer a mobile Learn to Row option. This is a trailer loaded with easy-to-assemble, stable boats which can be set up and ready to go in 10 minutes of arriving on site. It means that young people have to travel for far less time than they would normally: 'Rowing comes to you, rather than you going to row.' LYR has even set up a project to deliver rowing on one of the most iconic stretches of water in London, the Serpentine Lake in Hyde Park.

Competitions over the Internet have provided a further dimension – and also some excellent publicity. At the Xchanging Oxford and Cambridge Boat Race, LYR ran an indoor rowing competition on the finish line of the race itself. Young people in London raced against young people in Chicago, members of the Chicago Training Centre. They raced on line in real time through the RowPro software. It allowed the young people to see and chat to each other via webcams in-between races, and as people in Chicago watched the Boat Race on satellite TV, they also got to see the same young people thay had just raced against onscreen celebrating in the background as the winning crew crossed the line in front of more than 500 million viewers worldwide.

Matt and his team have clear advice for anyone wanting to develop a similar project:

- Be professional in every aspect. There are many sports organisations wanting to attract young people. Good marketing and publicity is essential. Sell the benefits.
- Provide a support structure for participating schools and youth clubs – and resources that are effective in enabling them to deliver their goals. For example, schools are asked to put aside £1200 each year so that they can replace the loan ergometers at the end of the project. They will be given the opportunity to buy refurbished ones.

- Participation has to be made easy for teachers. They are busy and have lots of pressures on them. One example of support is laminated lesson plans that correspond to the number of club sessions in a term, and also to ensure that they match what is required in the syllabus, making it easy for the schools to get involved. The teachers must also be able to see the benefits of the inputs they make.
- If you want to engage youth clubs, do not fall into the trap of using the same resources: young people go to a youth club because they want to, they go to school because they have to – there is a difference!
- There has to be relevant and obvious pathways of development to both competitions and to rowing on water.
- The sessions need to be engaging, challenging and fun.

These are good points for UK clubs that are increasingly under pressure from local councils to improve their involvement in the community.

REFERENCES

Anderson, M. E., Bruce, C. R., Fraser, S. F., Stepto, N. K., Klein, R., Hopkins, W. G., et al. (2000). Improved 2000-meter rowing performance in competitive oarswomen after caffeine ingestion. *Int J Sport Nutr Exerc Metab, 10*(4), 464–475.

Baghurst, T., Thierry, G., & Holder, T. (2004). Evidence for a relationship between attentional styles and effective cognitive strategies during performance. *Athl Insight, 6*(1), 36–51.

Baguet, A., Bourgois, J., Vanhee, L., Achten, E., & Derave, W. (2010). Important role of muscle carnosine in rowing performance. *J Appl Physiol, 109*(4), 1096–1101.

Bompa, T. O. (1994). *Periodization: Theory and Methodology of Training* (4th ed.). Champaign, IL: Human Kinetics.

Bourdin, M., Messonnier, L., Hager, J. P., & Lacour, J. R. (2004). Peak power output predicts rowing ergometer performance in elite male rowers. *Int J Sports Med, 25*(5), 368–373.

Bruce, C. R., Anderson, M. E., Fraser, S. F., Stepto, N. K., Klein, R., Hopkins, W. G., et al. (2000). Enhancement of 2000-m rowing performance after caffeine ingestion. *Med Sci Sports Exerc, 32*(11), 1958–1963.

Burge, C. M., Carey, M. F., & Payne, W. R. (1993). Rowing performance, fluid balance, and metabolic function following dehydration and rehydration. *Med Sci Sports Exerc, 25*(12), 1358–1364.

Burke, L. (2007). *Practical Sports Nutrition*. Leeds: Human Kinetics.

Cosgrove, M. J., Wilson, J., Watt, D., & Grant, S. F. (1999). The relationship between selected physiological variables of rowers and rowing performance as determined by a 2000 m ergometer test. *J Sports Sci, 17*(11), 845–852.

Coyle, E. F. (1999). Physiological determinants of endurance exercise performance. *J Sci Med Sport, 2*(3), 181–189.

Coyle, E. F. (2005). Improved muscular efficiency displayed as Tour de France champion matures. *J Appl Physiol, 98*(6), 2191–2196.

Coyle, E. F., Sidossis, L. S., Horowitz, J. F., & Beltz, J. D. (1992). Cycling efficiency is related to the percentage of type I muscle fibers. *Med Sci Sports Exerc, 24*(7), 782–788.

Hagerman, F. C. (1984). Applied physiology of rowing. *Sports Med, 1*(4), 303–326.

Hagerman, F. C. (1994). Physiology and nutrition for rowing. In D. R. Lamb, H. G. Knuttgen & R. Murray (Eds.), *Perspectives in Exercise Science and Sports Medicine* (Vol. 7, pp. 221–302). Carmel, IN: Quaker.

Hardman, A. E., & Stensel, D. J. (2009). *Physical Activity and Health: The Evidence Explained* (2nd ed.). London: Routledge.

Holsgaard-Larsen, A., & Jensen, K. (2010). Ergometer rowing with and without slides. *Int J Sports Med, 31*(12), 870–874.

Horowitz, J. F., Sidossis, L. S., & Coyle, E. F. (1994). High efficiency of type I muscle fibers improves performance. *Int J Sports Med, 15*(3), 152–157.

Ingham, S. A., Whyte, G. P., Jones, K., & Nevill, A. M. (2002). Determinants of 2,000 m rowing ergometer performance in elite rowers. *Eur J Appl Physiol, 88*(3), 243–246.

Josse, A. R., Tang, J. E., Tarnopolsky, M. A., & Phillips, S. M. (2010). Body composition and strength changes in women with milk and resistance exercise. *Med Sci Sports Exerc, 42*(6), 1122–1130.

Lakomy, H. K., & Lakomy, J. (1993). Estimation of maximum oxygen uptake from submaximal exercise on a Concept II rowing ergometer. *J Sports Sci, 11*(3), 227–232.

Lander, P. J., Butterly, R. J., & Edwards, A. M. (2009). Self-paced exercise is less physically challenging than enforced constant pace exercise of the same intensity: Influence of complex central metabolic control. *Br J Sports Med, 43*(10), 789–795.

Lawton, T. W., Cronin, J. B., & McGuigan, M. R. Strength testing and training of rowers: A review. *Sports Med, 41*(5), 413–432.

Lay, B. S., Sparrow, W. A., Hughes, K. M., & O'Dwyer, N. J. (2002). Practice effects on coordination and control, metabolic energy expenditure, and muscle activation. *Hum Mov Sci, 21*(5-6), 807–830.

Maestu, J., Jurimae, J., & Jurimae, T. (2005). Monitoring of performance and training in rowing. *Sports Med, 35*(7), 597–617.

Mahler, D. A., Hunter, B., Lentine, T., & Ward, J. (1991). Locomotor-respiratory coupling develops in novice female rowers with training. *Med Sci Sports Exerc, 23*(12), 1362–1366.

Mahler, D. A., Shuhart, C. R., Brew, E., & Stukel, T. A. (1991). Ventilatory responses and entrainment of breathing during rowing. *Med Sci Sports Exerc, 23*(2), 186–192.

Mahony, N., Donne, B., & O'Brien, M. (1999). A comparison of physiological responses to rowing on friction-loaded and air-braked ergometers. *J Sports Sci, 17*(2), 143–149.

McNaughton, L., & Cedaro, R. (1991). The effect of sodium bicarbonate on rowing ergometer performance in elite rowers. *The Aust J Sci Med Sport, 23*(3), 66–69.

Mikulic, P., Smoljanovic, T., Bojanic, I., Hannafin, J. A., & Matkovic, B. R. (2009). Relationship between 2000-m rowing ergometer performance times and World Rowing Championships rankings in elite-standard rowers. *J Sports Sci, 27*(9), 907–913.

Mikulic, P., Smoljanovic, T., Bojanic, I., Hannafin, J., & Pedisic, Z. (2009). Does 2000-m rowing ergometer performance time correlate with final rankings at the World Junior Rowing Championship? A case study of 398 elite junior rowers. *J Sports Sci, 27*(4), 361–366.

NHS (2010). *Health Survey for England 2008: Physical Activity and Fitness 2008*: Health and Social Care Information Centre.

Nieman, D. C., Davis, J. M., Henson, D. A., Gross, S. J., Dumke, C. L., Utter, A. C., et al. (2005). Muscle cytokine mRNA changes after 2.5 h of cycling: influence of carbohydrate. *Med Sci Sports Exerc, 37*(8), 1283–1290.

Nieman, D. C., Nehlsen-Cannarella, S. L., Fagoaga, O. R., Henson, D. A., Shannon, M., Davis, J. M., et al. (1999). Immune response to two hours of rowing in elite female rowers. *Int J Sports Med, 20*(7), 476–481.

Noakes, T. D. (2003). *Lore of Running* (4th ed.). Leeds: Human Kinetics.

Pollock, M. L., Gaesser, G. A., Butcher, J. D., Despres, J., Dishman, R. K., Franklin, B. A., et al. (1998). American College of Sports Medicine Position Stand. The recommended quantity and quality of exercise for developing and maintaining cardiorespiratory and muscular fitness, and flexibility in healthy adults. *Med Sci Sports Exerc, 30*(6), 975–991.

Rendi, M., Szabo, A., & Szabo, T. (2008). Performance enhancement with music in rowing sprint. *Sport Psychol, 22*(2), 175–182.

Rhodes, R. E., Warburton, D. E., & Murray, H. (2009). Characteristics of physical activity guidelines and their effect on adherence: A review of randomized trials. *Sports Med, 39*(5), 355–375.

Rice, T. (2009). *Information for Athletes, Head Coaches, Coaches and Scientists Protocol: Distance-Power Ergometer Testing.* Canberra: Australian Institute of Sport.

Rossiter, H. B., Cannell, E. R., & Jakeman, P. M. (1996). The effect of oral creatine supplementation on the 1000-m performance of competitive rowers. *J Sports Sci, 14*(2), 175–179.

Sawka, M. N., Burke, L. M., Eichner, E. R., Maughan, R. J., Montain, S. J., & Stachenfeld, N. S. (2007). American College of Sports Medicine position stand. Exercise and fluid replacement. *Med Sci Sports Exerc, 39*(2), 377–390.

Schabort, E. J., Hawley, J. A., Hopkins, W. G., & Blum, H. (1999). High reliability of performance of well-trained rowers on a rowing ergometer. *J Sports Sci, 17*(8), 627–632.

Scott, L. M., Scott, D., Bedic, S. P., & Dowd, J. (1999). The effect of associative and dissociative strategies on rowing ergometer performance. Mar 1999. *Sport Psychol, 13*(1), 57–68.

Secher, N. H. (1993). Physiological and biomechanical aspects of rowing. Implications for training. *Sports Med, 15*(1), 24–42.

Secher, N. H., & Vaage, O. (1983). Rowing performance, a mathematical model based on analysis of body dimensions as exemplified by body weight. *Eur J Appl Physiol Occup Physiol, 52*(1), 88–93.

Silva, J. M., & Appelbaum, M. I. (1989). Association-dissociation patterns of United States Olympic Marathon Trial contestants. *Cognitive Ther Res, 13*(2), 57–68.

Simonsen, J. C., Sherman, W. M., Lamb, D. R., Dernbach, A. R., Doyle, J. A., & Strauss, R. (1991). Dietary carbohydrate, muscle glycogen, and power output during rowing training. *J Appl Physiol, 70*(4), 1500–1505.

Singh, M., & Das, R. R. Zinc for the common cold. *Cochrane Database Syst Rev, 2,* CD001364.

Skinner, T. L., Jenkins, D. G., Coombes, J. S., Taaffe, D. R., & Leveritt, M. D. Dose response of caffeine on 2000-m rowing performance. *Med Sci Sports Exerc, 42*(3), 571–576.

Slater, G. J., Rice, A. J., Sharpe, K., Mujika, I., Jenkins, D., & Hahn, A. G. (2005). Body-mass management of Australian lightweight rowers prior to and during competition. *Med Sci Sports Exerc, 37*(5), 860–866.

Slater, G. J., Rice, A. J., Sharpe, K., Tanner, R., Jenkins, D., Gore, C. J., et al. (2005). Impact of acute weight loss and/or thermal stress on rowing ergometer performance. *Med Sci Sports Exerc, 37*(8), 1387–1394.

Slater, G., Rice, A. J., Tanner, R., Sharpe, K., Gore, C. J., Jenkins, D. G., et al. (2006). Acute weight loss followed by an aggressive nutritional recovery strategy has little impact on on-water rowing performance. *Br J Sports Med, 40*(1), 55–59.

Smith, R. M., & Spinks, W. L. (1995). Discriminant analysis of biomechanical differences between novice, good and elite rowers. *J Sports Sci, 13*(5), 377–385.

Soper, C., & Hume, P. A. (2004). Reliability of power output during rowing changes with ergometer type and race distance. *Sports Biomech, 3*(2), 237–248.

Steinacker, J. M., Both, M., & Whipp, B. J. (1993). Pulmonary mechanics and entrainment of respiration and stroke rate during rowing. *Int J Sports Med, 14 Suppl 1*, S15–19.

Syrotuik, D. G., Game, A. B., Gillies, E. M., & Bell, G. J. (2001). Effects of creatine monohydrate supplementation during combined strength and high intensity rowing training on performance. *Can J Appl Physiol, 26*(6), 527–542.

Tenenbaum, G., & Connolly, C. T. (2008). Attention allocation under varied workload and effort perception in rowers. *Psychol Sport Exerc, 9*(5), 704–717.

USDHHS. (2008a). 2008 Physical Activity Guidelines for Americans [Electronic Version]. Retrieved April 11, 2011 from http://www.health.gov/paguidelines/.

USDHHS. (2008b). US Physical Activity Statistics. Retrieved April 15, 2011 from http://apps.nccd.cdc.gov/PASurveillance/StateSumResultV.asp?CI=&Year=2007&State=0

Vinther, A., Alkjaer, T., Kanstrup, I. L., Zerahn, B., Ekdahl, C., Jensen, K., et al. (2011). Neuromuscular activity and force production during slide-based and stationary ergometer rowing. *Br J Sports Med, 45*(4), 381–382.

Vogler, A. J., Rice, A. J., & Gore, C. J. (2010). Physiological responses to ergometer and on-water incremental rowing tests. *Int J Sports Physiol Perform, 5*(3), 342–358.

Vogler, A. J., Rice, A. J., & Withers, R. T. (2007). Physiological responses to exercise on different models of the concept II rowing ergometer. *Int J Sports Physiol Perform, 2*(4), 360–370.

Volianitis, S., McConnell, A. K., Koutedakis, Y., McNaughton, L., Backx, K., & Jones, D. A. (2001). Inspiratory muscle training improves rowing performance. *Med Sci Sports Exerc, 33*(5), 803–809.

Wilmore, J. H., & Costill, D. L. (2004). *Physiology of Sport and Exercise* (3rd ed.). Leeds: Human Kinetics.

INDEX

ventilation 40–1
volume of exercise 57, 59–60

water rower system 9
websites 68
weight-adjusted scoring 121–3
weight, bearing on ability of 37–8
weight loss 124–5, 131, 133–6
    benefits of indoor rowing to 66–7
World Indoor Rowing Championships vii, 4